Infection Control

FOR

Prehospital Care Providers

Second Edition

Lynn Zimmerman, R.N., B.S.N., M.Ed.

Mary Neuman, R.N., B.S.N.

Deb Jurewicz, R.N., EMT-P

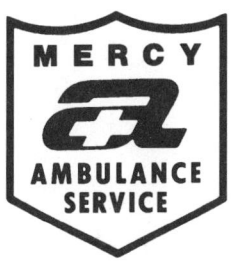

Published by
Mercy Ambulance
Grand Rapids, Michigan

Copyright 1993 Mercy Ambulance

All Rights Reserved

Library of Congress Catalog Card Number: 93-77350
ISBN – 0-9615819-1-3

Revised Edition of: Infection Control Procedures For Prehospital Care Providers, 1985

Additional copies may be obtained by writing to:
Mercy Ambulance
517 S. Division
Grand Rapids, Michigan 49503

This book is dedicated to all of the men and women who have chosen to serve in the Emergency Medical Services and Public Safety professions. To keep them safe and well so they will continue to be there when we need them.

ACKNOWLEDGMENTS

TO

The following individuals who gave of their time and expertise in assisting the authors with this work:

Professional reviewers:

Paul Farr, M.D. – Internist – specializing in gastrointestinal diseases

David Baumgartner, M.D. – Specialist in Infectious Diseases

Deborah Rose, Ph.D – Psychologist

Carolyn Douma, M.Ed. – Reading Specialist

The following individuals for their invaluable assistance in publishing this text.

Joyce Hoopfer
Typist

Mary Salamone
Illustrations/Design

Helga Bidwell/Bidwell Consulting
Composition

Erdmans Printing Company
Printer

Mercy Ambulance
Publisher

Proceeds from the sale of this book
will be donated to the
R.D. Brady Foundation for Prehospital Research

Infection Control
for
Prehospital Care Providers

TABLE OF CONTENTS

Preface 11
Introduction by David Baumgartner, M.D. 13

CHAPTER 1   How Diseases Are Spread 15

CHAPTER 2   General Isolation Guidelines 19
    General Isolation Instructions 21
    Universal Precautions 23
    Barrier Techniques 25
    Isolation Categories 33
        Category Specific Isolation Guidelines 33
        Symptom Specific Isolation Guidelines 45
        Disease Specific Isolation Guidelines 49
    Preparing for Transport 75

CHAPTER 3   Employee Exposure & Illness 77
    Blood Borne Pathogens 81
        A.   AIDS 81
        B.   Hepatitis B 84
            Delta Hepatitis 86
            Hepatitis C 86
            Non-A, Non-B Hepatitis 87
        C.   Babesiosis 87
        D.   Brucellosis 88
        E.   Colorado Tick Fever (Arboviral) 89
        F.   Creutzfeldt-Jakob 90
        G.   Hemorrhagic Fever 91
        H.   HTLV 92
        I.   Leptospirosis 92
        J.   Malaria 93
        K.   Syphilis 94
        L.   Relapsing Fever 95
    Campylobacter 96
    Childhood 96
        A.   Chickenpox 96
        B.   Measles 97
        C.   Mumps 97
        D.   Rubella 98
        E.   Pertussis 99
    Common Colds 99
    Conjunctivitis 100
    CMV 101

CHAPTER 3 (Continued)
- Diphtheria 101
- Gastrointestinal Illnesses 101
- Giardia Lamblia 102
- Hepatitis Non-Blood Borne 102
  - A. Hepatitis A & E 102
- Herpes Simplex 103
- Meninigitis 104
  - A. Meningococcal 104
  - B. H Flu 105
- Plague 105
  - A. Bubonic and Pneumonic 105
- Pneumonia 106
- Rabies 106
- Salmonella 107
- Scabies 107
- Shigella 108
- Staph Aureus 108
- Strep Throat 109
- Tetanus 109
- Tuberculosis 110
- Wound Infection 111
- Blood Exposure Algorithm 112
- Special Section: 115
  - Employees with chronic or life-threatening illnesses. 115
  - American Ambulance Association's Position Statement 118
- Case Study 121

CHAPTER 4 Cleaning & Disinfection 123
- Disposable Supplies and Equipment 125
- Regulated Waste 125
- Non-disposable Equipment & Work Surfaces 127
- Laundry/Linens 128
- Care of Contaminated Articles 129
- Cleaning of Contaminated Articles 129

CHAPTER 5 Exposure Control Plan "The OSHA Rule" 137
- Summary of the Bloodborne Pathogen Standard 139
- Case Study 153

CHAPTER 6 Training & Education 155
- Infection Control - General 157
- Exposure Control Plans & Bloodborne Pathogens 159
- Tuberculosis 187
- Case Study 191

CHAPTER 7 Recordkeeping 193

CHAPTER 8	QA Surveillance & Monitoring	205
CHAPTER 9	Employee Health & Hygiene Policies & Procedures	211
CHAPTER 10	Disaster Implications	223
ABBREVIATIONS		229
GLOSSARY		231
FOOTNOTES		239
BIBLIOGRAPHY		241
INDEX		245

PREFACE

In the world of emergency prehospital medicine, infectious diseases do not have a lot of visibility, nor do they demand a great deal of attention. Trauma and cardiac cases are far more volatile, and carry with them a sense of urgency not often seen with communicable disease. Our attitudes also reflect a belief that infectious diseases are only a problem in developing Third World countries or that we have vaccines that eliminate any serious problem.

Our complacency could be fatal to our patients, our families, and ourselves if it leads us to ignore proper infection control procedures and by doing so, contribute to the spread of disease.

Disease-causing viruses and bacteria are highly mobile and adaptable. Prehospital care givers deal not only with those diseases most commonly found in the United States, but more and more can expect to encounter strains brought into this country by refugees and immigrants, vacation travelers, animals and vegetation.

Infectious diseases exist which are capable of afflicting or killing hundreds of thousands of people. Yesterday's bubonic plague and cholera are today's AIDS, Hepatitis B. Newspaper accounts highlight measles outbreaks on college campuses, reoccurrence of poliomyelitis in former victims, and the resurgence of Tuberculosis.

Emergency Medical Service (EMS) providers need to be concerned, and they need to act. Effective infection control depends more on effort and common sense than on money or high-tech equipment.

INTRODUCTION

by
David Baumgartner, M.D.

Historically, the prehospital care provider has been a weak link in infection control. This has resulted not from a lack of concern on the part of providers but from the fact that prehospital care providers cannot control the conditions under which they find patients, nor in most cases can they predict a patient's likelihood of transmitting infection. Furthermore, there remain many misconceptions regarding infection control among health care providers in general. On the other hand, the intense publicity surrounding bloodborne diseases such as Human Immunodeficiency Virus (HIV) as well as the recognition of other transmittable diseases such as Hepatitis C have focused our efforts on infection control as never before. What was once an abstraction to many health care workers has now become a topic of vital interest.

Traditional literature on infection control has often been silent on many issues of specific concern to the prehospital care provider. The interest that the previous edition of this book elicited speaks to the need for a work of this effort. While there is still much to be learned from hospital-based infection control, this edition includes new information that has been established by experience during the AIDS epidemic as well as focusing on newer guidelines from the Centers for Disease Control (CDC). In addition, this edition reflects the policies that must be carried out to comply with the new OSHA regulations regarding prevention of transmission of infectious agents in the work place.

The purpose of this manual is to establish guidelines for infection control in the prehospital setting. Because conditions in the prehospital environment fluctuate widely, the guidelines in this manual are more rigid than might be found in an institution.

The focus for the prehospital provider must be on:
- ELIMINATION, wherever possible, of the SOURCES of disease which can be controlled by adequate cleansing and disinfection of vehicles and equipment.
- PREVENTION of TRANSMISSION of disease by adequate barrier precautions utilizing gloves, gowns, masks and goggles where appropriate.
- REDUCTION in SUSCEPTIBILITY to infection by maintaining good general health, hygiene, and getting immunizations done routinely.

A section of the book has been developed to offer suggestions for personnel health and hygiene policies. It will be necessary for a provider to completely review this manual and in conjunction with their medical advisors adopt those sections of the personnel practices that reflect protocols and policies for their area.

This is a rapidly changing area as new infectious agents are discovered, new immunizations become available and changing state and federal regulations place a greater burden on the employer to prevent transmission of infection. Therefore, users of this manual must periodically review and update their information. One of the truisms of infection control is that odd circumstances will occur that just don't seem to be covered by written policies. For that reason, there is no replacement for establishing a relationship with an individual who has experience as an infection control practitioner. Such individuals may be infection control or employee health nurses, infectious disease physicians or physicians with experience in industrial health. What they all share is a commitment to the prevention of infection in the work setting and an ability to problem shoot, anticipate problems, and keep up with the rapidly changing infection control scene. Such resources are ignored at one's own risk.

CHAPTER ONE

How Diseases Are Spread

NOTES

How Diseases Are Spread

There are three elements essential to the spread of disease:

I. A source of infection
II. A means of transmission
III. A susceptible host

If any of the three elements are eliminated,
an infection cannot be communicated.

I. SOURCE

A source of infecting organisms may be either a living thing or an inanimate object. People serve as a common source of infections: patients, family members, bystanders, and employees. These individuals harbor many micro-organisms, some of which can become or are disease producing. These individuals may have active disease, may be in the incubation period of the disease (the time when they are capable of spreading infection but have no or few symptoms of the disease itself), or they may be carriers of disease. In some situations a person's own normal flora (micro-organisms that inhabit the body without producing disease normally) may cause disease.

Other living organisms may serve as sources of infection, including animals, insects, etc. However, these are of lesser consequence for most prehospital care providers in the United States.

Inanimate objects can become contaminated and thus serve as a source of infection. Most often these are objects used by infectious patients, such as water glasses, clothing, bed linens, dressings, etc. Obviously, items used by prehospital care providers can become contaminated in the same manner and must be decontaminated prior to reusing.

II. TRANSMISSION OF DISEASES

Disease are transmitted via one of four routes:
1. Contact
    A. Direct contact requires direct physical contact between an infected person and a susceptible host. Example: Herpes Simplex.
    B. Indirect contact can occur when an infected person contaminates an inanimate object and a susceptible host comes in contact with the contaminated object. Example: Chickenpox.
    C. Droplet contact is the spread of infection through droplets sprayed from an infected person's mouth and/or nose. This can occur with coughing, sneezing, or even talking. This is considered a contact means of transmission because droplet spread requires close proximity, within three feet. At any greater distances, the droplets will normally fall harmlessly to the floor and dry up, thus posing no further threat. Example: Meningococcal Meningitis

2. Vehicles

Diseases that are transmitted by vehicles are spread by one of the following mediums:
A. Food
B. Water
C. Drugs
D. Blood

Example: Salmonella or Hepatitis.

3. Airborne

Diseases that can be transmitted via airborne route are usually organisms that are suspended in the air as droplet nuclei or on dust particles. Example: Tuberculosis.

4. Vectorborne

The vectorborne route requires the involvement of an intermediate host, such as a fly, mosquito, tick or flea. These vectors can transmit the infection through simple mechanical means; that is, a micro-organism will attach itself to the legs or the body of the vector and then allow the vector to deposit the micro-organism on the next object or susceptible host with which it comes in contact. The second mechanism of transmission via vectors is termed biological. In this example the micro-organism will traditionally go through some life cycle change while inhabiting the body of the intermediate host. The intermediate host will then transmit this changed micro-organism to a susceptible host. Examples: Rocky Mountain Spotted Fever, Colorado Tick Fever, Bubonic Plague and Malaria.

III. SUSCEPTIBLE HOST

The third and final element that is essential for the spread of diseases is a susceptible host. A susceptible host is any person or animal that is capable of becoming infected with the disease being transmitted. There are many things that can increase or decrease a person's susceptibility to a specific infection, including but not limited to the degree of general good health the person enjoys, personal hygiene practices, active or passive immunizations, adequate nutrition, and the presence of any concurrent illness or shock to the body. In addition, there are several debilitating conditions that may contribute to increasing the susceptibility of a person to disease. These include certain immunosuppressant diseases such as HIV/AIDS, cancer, leukemia and aplastic anemia. Additionally, certain drugs will act to suppress immune capabilities including cortico-steroids and many of the anti-cancer chemotherapeutic drugs. Age can also be a factor, with the very young and the very old more susceptible to infections.

Chapter Two

General Isolation Guidlines

- **General Isolation Instructions**
- **Universal Precautions**
- **Barrier Techniques**
- **Isolation Categories**
- **Preparing for Transport**

Notes

General Isolation Instructions

ALL EMPLOYEES ARE EXPECTED TO:

1. Be familiar with the contents of the infection control manual and Exposure Control Plan.
2. Instruct patients to cover mouth with tissue when coughing.
3. Assure that disposable masks are worn when indicated. Masks shall cover the mouth and nose, and be changed every half hour or as they become moisture laden. Masks shall be discarded into the appropriate trash container. Masks shall not be allowed to be lowered around the neck and reused.
4. Wear the designated impervious outerwear (gowns, aprons, jumpsuits) when indicated. Disposable outerwear shall be discarded in an appropriately labelled biohazard bag.
5. Wear gloves of the disposable, single-use type. Gloves will be discarded into appropriate trash containers after use.
6. Wash hands and arms thoroughly, using designated hand disinfectant before and after transporting a patient, after removing personal protective equipment (PPE), before entering cab of vehicle and before eating, drinking, smoking or applying lip balm or make-up.
7. Any contaminated instruments, equipment, etc., are to be cleaned of visible soil and decontaminated prior to reuse.
8. Discard all disposable items in appropriate container. Contaminated items should be placed in the appropriately labelled biohazard container.
9. If working in conjunction with a cooperating hospital, be thoroughly familiar with that hospital's infection control standards.

NOTES

UNIVERSAL PRECAUTIONS

It is safe to assume that everyone has the potential for an infectious disease and our actions in caring for our patients should be directed toward that assumption. Universal Precautions provide us with this concept. The word Universal by itself means applicable or common to all purposes, a universal remedy. Precaution means an action taken in advance to protect against possible danger or failure; a safeguard. When both words are placed together, they mean a process that applies to everyone who may be placed in situations that might expose them to blood or body fluids.

Body fluids include amniotic fluid, pericardial fluid, peritoneal fluid, pleural fluid, synovial fluid, CSF, semen and vaginal secretions or any body fluid with visible blood. However, when EMS and public safety workers encounter body fluids under uncontrolled, emergency circumstances, in which differentiation between fluid types is difficult, if not impossible, they should treat all body fluids as potentially hazardous.

In August, 1987, the Centers for Disease Control (CDC) issued guidelines designed to minimize the risk of bloodborne pathogens in health care settings. These guidelines have come to be called Universal Precautions. The intent of these precautions is clear. All patients have the potential to harbor bloodborne pathogens; therefore blood and body fluids from all patients should be considered hazardous.

Many health care professionals feel infection control procedures are very cumbersome to follow. EMS workers complain about the time it takes to put on the PPE, that the garments were not designed for prehospital and thus interfere with dexterity, and they are uncomfortable.

None of the above reasons are good enough reasons to chance the risk of exposure to life threatening illnesses. All health care workers need to be constantly evaluating their techniques as they relate to infection control.

Table 2.1 Summary of Universal Precautions and Recommendations

Handwashing should be performed before and after patient contact, immediately if hands are contaminated with blood or other body fluids, and after removing gloves.

Gloves should be worn when soiling of the hands with blood or body fluids is likely.

Gowns are generally not indicated; however, gowns should be worn if soiling of exposed skin or clothing is likely.

Masks are generally not indicated; however, masks should be worn when splashing or splattering of blood or other body fluids is likely. A mask alone is not sufficient protection but should be worn in combination with protective eyewear.

Protective eyewear is usually not indicated; however, protective eyewear should be worn when splashing or splattering of blood or other body fluids is likely. Personal eyewear often offers adequate protection. Eyewear should always be worn with a mask (see above).

A private room is generally not indicated; however, a patient should be placed in a private room if hygienic practices are poor or if the environment is likely to be soiled with blood or body fluids.

Patients may receive regular food service on reusable dishes; no special precautions are indicated for meal service.

Reusable, contaminated equipment should be cleaned of visible organic material, placed in an impervious container and returned to central hospital supply for decontamination and reprocessing.

Contaminated needles and other disposable sharp objects should be handled carefully. Used needles should never be bent, clipped, or recapped. Contaminated sharp objects should be discarded immediately after use into a puncture-resistant container designed for this purpose. Needle containers should not be overfilled; containers should be sealed and discarded when two-thirds to three-fourths full.

To minimize the risks for exchange of body fluids, pocket masks or mechanical ventilation devices should be readily available in areas in which resuscitation procedures are likely to be needed.

Spills of blood or blood-containing body fluids should be cleaned up by: first, donning gloves (and other barriers if indicated); second, wiping up excess material with disposable towels; third, cleansing with soap and water; and fourth, disinfecting with a dilute solution (1:100 for smooth surfaces; 1:10 for porous surfaces) of household bleach (sodium hypochlorite) and water. Diluted bleach solution should be no more than 24 hours old. Large spills or spills containing broken glass or sharp objects should be covered with disposable towels; second, saturated with 1:10 bleach solution and allowed to stand for at least 10 minutes; and third, cleaned up as outlined above.

Health care workers who have open lesions, dermatitis, etc., should refrain from direct patient care and from directly handling contaminated equipment. Such employees should be evaluated by employee health services or by a private physician to assess fitness for duty.

Compliance with these precautions is the responsibility of the health care employer. Employers must provide: orientation, training and continuing education for all health care workers, along with adequate barriers and supplies. Employers are required to monitor compliance with universal precautions. Employers should develop mechanisms for counseling and retraining of noncompliant employees and should develop appropriate disciplinary action for repeatedly noncompliant employees.

(Modified from Centers for Disease Control)

BARRIER TECHNIQUES

GLOVING TECHNIQUE:

TO GLOVE:

A. Wash hands.
B. Place disposable gloves over hands.
C. Pull gloves over the cuffs of the gown, if gown is worn.

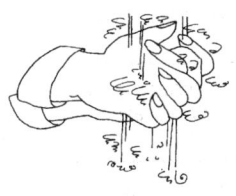 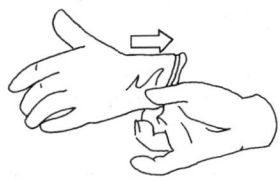 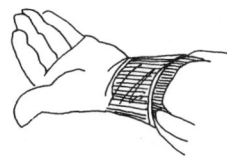

TO REMOVE GLOVES:

A. Place two fingers 1/2 inch from top of glove.
B. Pull top of glove over the fingers.
C. Pull over the hand.
D. Pull the other glove down with the covered hand.

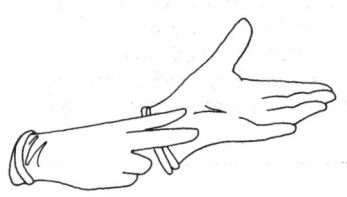 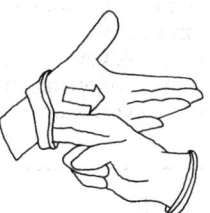 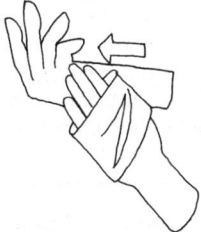

TO REMOVE GLOVES: (Continued)

E. Dispose of gloves in appropriate receptacle.
F. Wash hands and forearms at handwashing facility or before leaving patient's room or Emergency Department.

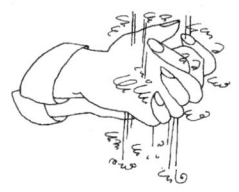

MASK & EYE PROTECTION OR FACE SHIELD TECHNIQUES:

TO MASK:

A. Place disposable mask over mouth and nose.
B. Pinch metal section on mask to secure, if applicable; some masks must be spread to fit properly.
C. Change mask every half hour or anytime it becomes moisture laden on the inside.
D. Never lower mask around neck and then reuse.

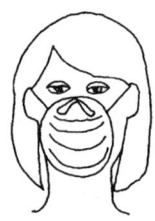 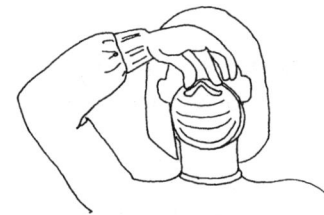

TO REMOVE MASK:

A. Remove mask by rubber bands or ties only.
B. Discard in an appropriate waste container or isolation bag in isolation room or Emergency Department.
C. Wash hands and forearms at handwashing facility or before leaving patient's room or Emergency Department.

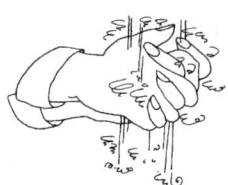

General Isolation Guidelines

EYE PROTECTION

TO PUT ON EYE PROTECTION:

A. Select appropriate eye protection that includes shielding from front, sides and top. Goggles, safety glasses with side and top shields as well as full face shields are all acceptable. Prescription glasses are acceptable if side and top shielding are added.
B. Place securely on face.

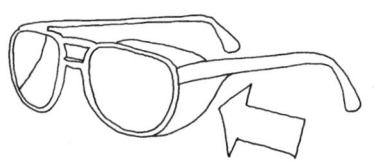

TO REMOVE EYE PROTECTION:

A. Remove eye protection with gloved hands, avoiding touching your face or head with your hand.
B. Decontaminate eyewear prior to reusing or dispose if appropriate.

FACESHIELD

TO APPLY:

A. Place faceshield on over mouth, nose and eyes.
B. Elastic bands are secured behind ears or helmet style is placed around head.

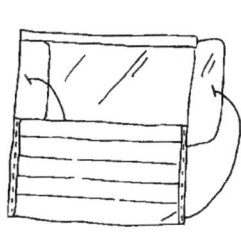 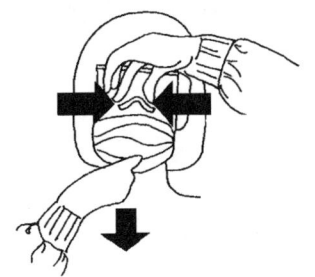 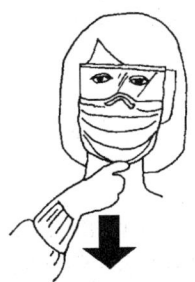

TO REMOVE:

A. If disposable, remove by rubber bands only after removing gloves.
B. Discard in appropriate container.
C. If non-disposable, remove faceshield before removing gloves. Clean and disinfect prior to reusing.

MASK AND EYE PROTECTION OR FACE SHIELD

Mask and eye protection/face shield shall be worn while performing invasive techniques including IV therapy, suctioning, and intubation, or anytime there is an opportunity for blood or body fluids to be splashed, sprayed, or splattered.

OUTERWEAR PROTECTION TECHNIQUE

TO GOWN:

A. Remove watch and rings, pin inside your pocket, and roll uniform sleeves above elbow.
B. Use a clean gown each time.
C. Keep gown from touching the floor.
D. Tie neckbands, lap gown at back, and tie waist ties.

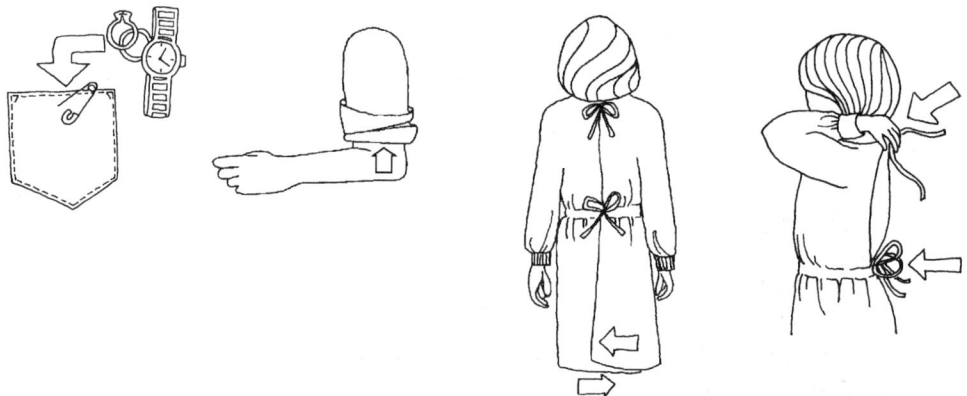

TO REMOVE A CONTAMINATED GOWN:

A. Wash hands.
B. Untie waist ties and neck ties.
C. Place two fingers inside of cuff and pull sleeve over the hand; avoid touching the sleeve on the outside.

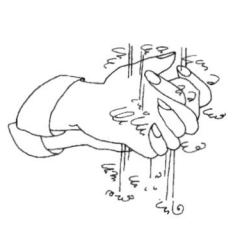 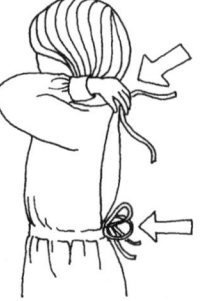 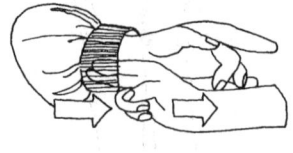

General Isolation Guidelines

TO REMOVE A CONTAMINATED GOWN: *(Continued)*

D. Pull the other sleeve down with the covered hand.
E. Remove gown, folding clean side out by matching shoulder seams, roll up and place in linen bag (if non-disposable) or contaminated trash bag (if disposable).
F. Wash hands and forearms at handwashing facility before leaving isolation room or Emergency Department.

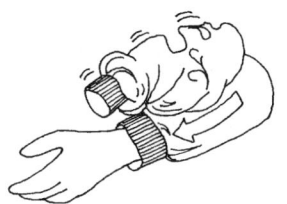 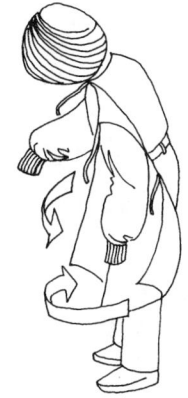 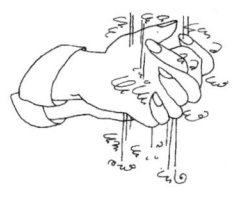

OTHER OUTERWEAR PROTECTION

TO SUIT A JUMPSUIT:

A. Step into leg portion of suit, insert arms and pull on over shoulders. Close by zipper or velcro closure.
B. If booties are included with suit, special care should be taken to avoid slipping and falling.

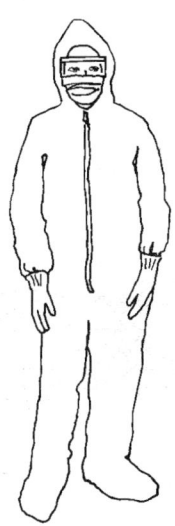

TO REMOVE A CONTAMINATED SUIT:

A. Unzip suit with gloved hands.
B. Remove gloves.
C. Pull arms out of suit being careful to only touch inside of suit with ungloved hands.
D. Step out of legs being careful not to contaminate personal clothing or skin.
E. Dispose of items in appropriate labelled container.
F. Wash hands.

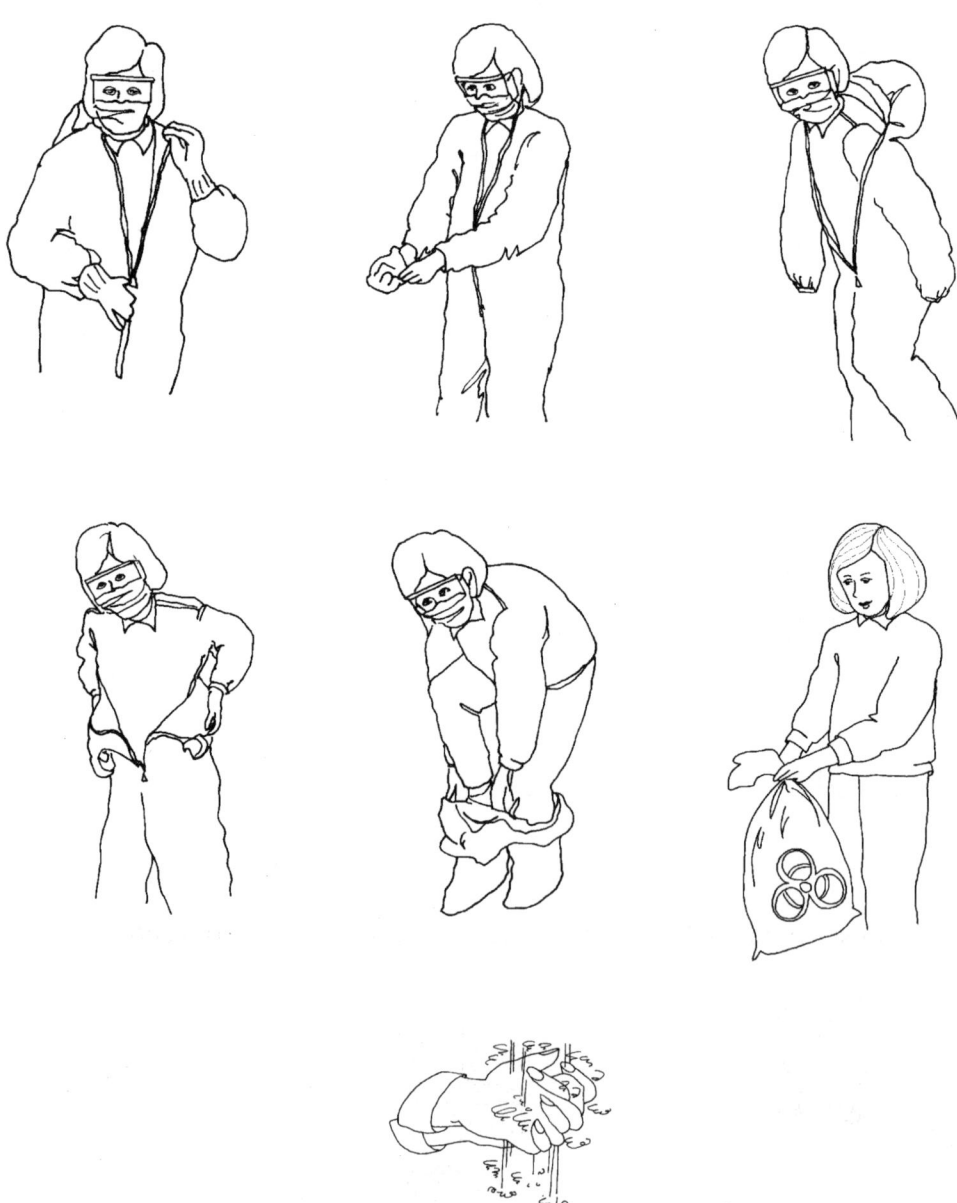

General Isolation Guidelines

SLEEVE PROTECTION

TO PUT ON:

A. Pull on sleeve protection, extending above elbow.
B. Put on gloves, being sure wrist section of glove pulls on over wrist area of sleeve protection.

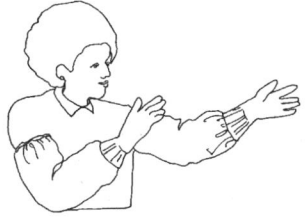

TO REMOVE:

A. Grab top outer portion of sleeve with gloved hand and pull down so that sleeve is turned inside out. Sleeve and glove should be removed simultaneously.
B. When removing second sleeve, unglloved hand should reach inside of top portion of sleeve, and remove sleeve by turning inside out. Again, sleeve and glove should be removed simultaneously.
C. Dispose of articles in appropriate labelled container.
D. Wash hands.

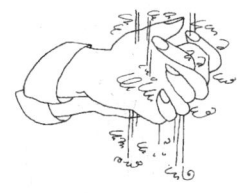

HEAD COVERINGS AND BOOTIES

TO PUT ON:

A. When putting on head coverings, be sure all hair is contained.
B. Caution should be taken once booties are on to avoid slipping and falling.

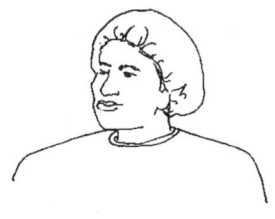 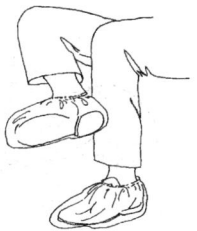

TO REMOVE:

A. Head coverings should be carefully removed to avoid contaminating hair/head.
B. Remove booties by pulling off with gloved hand.
C. Articles should be disposed of in appropriate labelled container.
D. Wash hands after removing PPE.

ISOLATION CATEGORIES

Category specific isolation techniques describes the seven types of isolation categories based on the mode of transmission of the various diseases. The seven types are:

- Strict Isolation*
- Contact Isolation*
- Respiratory Isolation*
- Tuberculosis (AFB) Isolation*
- Enteric Precautions
- Drainage/Secretion Precautions
- Blood/Body Fluid Precautions

For our purposes and because over-precautions are better than under-precautions especially in the uncontrolled EMS environment, *we have combined 'strict' and 'contact' into 'strict isolation' and have included tuberculosis with Respiratory Isolation. In this section, each of the isolation categories will be described including rationale, precautions to be used, and a listing of diseases requiring each isolation precaution category.

Along with the diseases, included in each category will be a listing of infective material. This is important to assist in determining whether or not contamination or transmission may have occurred. We will not be concerned about items or routes that are not applicable to that category/disease.

Strict isolation is indicated whenever a highly contagious infection is present and may be transmitted by contact and air.

Notes

Strict Isolation

- **MASKS** and **EYE WEAR** should be worn by all persons in ambulance.
- **OUTERWEAR** should be worn by all persons in ambulance.
- **GLOVES** should be worn by all persons in ambulance.
- **HANDS MUST BE WASHED AFTER REMOVING PPE, AFTER TOUCHING THE PATIENT OR POTENTIALLY CONTAMINATED ARTICLES AND BEFORE TAKING CARE OF ANOTHER PATIENT.**
- **ARTICLES** contaminated with infective material shall be discarded or decontaminated.
- **AMBULANCE** (patient compartment) must be disinfected and aired out after patient is removed.

*Diseases that require close contact for transmission to occur.

Diseases Requiring Strict Isolation

DISEASES	INFECTIVE MATERIAL
*Acute respiratory infections in infants and young children (croup, colds, bronchitis)	Respiratory secretions / Feces
*Conjunctivitis, gonococcal, in newborns	Purulent exudate or pus
Diphtheria	
cutaneous	Lesion secretions
pharyngeal	Respiratory secretions
*Endometritis (Group A strep)	Vaginal discharge
*Furunculosis (Staph in newborns)	Pus
Hemorrhagic Fever such as Lassa, Marburg, Ebola, Crimean–Congo Fever	Blood and Body fluids / Respiratory secretions
*Herpes Simplex, disseminated or primary	Lesion secretions
*Impetigo	Lesions
*Influenza in infants and young children	Respiratory secretions

DISEASES   INFECTIVE MATERIAL

Meningitis (unknown etiology) .... Blood and Body fluid
                                                                    Respiratory secretions

*Multiply-resistant bacteria, ... Feces, Urine and
infection or colonization .... Respiratory secretions

*Pediculosis (lice) .... Infested area

*Pharyngitis (sore throat) .... Respiratory secretions
in infants and young children

Plague, pneumonic .... Respiratory secretions

*Pneumonia, viral, ... Respiratory secretions
in infants and young children .... Feces

*Pneumonia, Staph Aureus or Group A Strep ... Respiratory secretions

*Rabies .... Respiratory secretions

Rubella .... Respiratory secretions
                                                                    Urine

*Scabies .... Infested area

*Scalded Skin Syndrome (Ritter's Disease) ...... Lesion drainage

*Skin, Wound or Burn infections, ... Pus
major, draining, not covered or
not contained by dressing

Smallpox .... Respiratory secretions
                                                                    Lesion secretions

*Vaccinia .... Lesion secretions

Varicella (Chickenpox) .... Respiratory secretions
                                                                    Lesion secretions

Varicella Zoster (Shingles), ... Lesion secretions
localized in immunocompromised
patient or disseminated .... Respiratory secretions

General Isolation Guidelines

RESPIRATORY ISOLATION

- **TIGHT FITTING MASK OR RESPIRATOR** should be worn by all persons in ambulance.* **EYE PROTECTION** also indicated.
- **GLOVES** may be used.
- **OUTERWEAR** not indicated.
- **HANDS MUST BE WASHED AFTER TOUCHING THE PATIENT OR POTENTIALLY CONTAMINATED ARTICLES AND BEFORE TAKING CARE OF ANOTHER PATIENT.**
- **ARTICLES** contaminated with infective materials must be decontaminated or discarded.
- **AMBULANCE** must be aired out after patient is removed. Any surfaces contaminated with infective material must be disinfected.

*If ambulance is of a type where the patient compartment and the driver compartment are separate, the driver of the vehicle may not be required to wear a mask.

DISEASES REQUIRING RESPIRATORY ISOLATION

DISEASES	INFECTIVE MATERIAL
Epiglottitis (H. flu)	Respiratory secretions
Erythema infectiosum (5th Disease)	Respiratory secretions
Measles (Rubeola)	Respiratory secretions
Meningitis	
H. flu	Respiratory secretions
Meningococcal	Respiratory secretions
Meningococcemia	Respiratory secretions
Mumps	Respiratory secretions
Pertussis (whooping cough)	Respiratory secretions
Pneumonia (H.flu in children)	Respiratory secretions
Tuberculosis (AFB isolation)	Respiratory secretions Droplet nuclei

NOTES

General Isolation Guidelines

BLOOD AND BODY FLUID PRECAUTIONS

- **MASKS AND EYEWEAR** are indicated if there is a possibility of the patient's blood or body fluids being sprayed or aerosolized, and subsequent contact with rescuer's mouth or face.
- **OUTERWEAR PROTECTION** should be work by all persons in ambulance if blood and/or body fluids may be present.
- **GLOVES** should be worn by all persons having patient contact if opportunity for contact with blood or body fluids may be present.
- **HANDS MUST BE WASHED AFTER REMOVING PPE, AFTER TOUCHING ANY PATIENT OR POTENTIALLY CONTAMINATED ARTICLES AND BEFORE TAKING CARE OF ANOTHER PATIENT.**
- **ARTICLES** contaminated with blood or body fluids must be discarded or decontaminated.

Any interior **AMBULANCE** surfaces contaminated with blood or body fluids must be cleaned up promptly with an Environmental Protection Agency (EPA) registered hospital disinfectant with label claim that it is tuberculocidal.

Care must be taken to avoid needle–stick and other percutaneous injuries. Used needles must not be recapped, bent or broken. They should be placed in a prominently labelled (biohazard), puncture-resistant container designated specifically for such disposal.

DISEASES REQUIRING BLOOD AND BODY FLUID PRECAUTIONS

DISEASES	INFECTIVE MATERIAL
Acquired Immunodeficiency Syndrome (AIDS)	Blood & Body fluids
Arthropodborne viral diseases (dengue, yellow & Colorado tick fever)	Blood
Babesiosis	Blood
Brucellosis	Blood & Body fluids, Pus
Creutzfeldt–Jakob Disease	Blood, Brain tissue and Spinal fluid
Hepatitis B (including Carrier States)	Blood & Body fluids

DISEASES	INFECTIVE MATERIAL
Hepatitis C	Blood & Body Fluids
Hepatitis, non-A non-B	Blood & Body fluids
Hemorrhagic Fevers	Blood & Body Fluids
Leptospirosis	Blood & Urine
Malaria	Blood
Rat-bite Fever	Blood
Relapsing Fever	Blood
Syphilis, primary & secondary	Lesion secretions & Blood

General Isolation Guidelines

DRAINAGE AND SECRETION PRECAUTIONS

- **OUTERWEAR PRTOECTION** should be worn by all persons who may have contact with infective material.
- **GLOVES** should be worn by all persons who may have contact with infective material.
- **MASKS** are not indicated.
- **AFTER REMOVING PPE, AFTER TOUCHING THE PATIENT OR POTENTIALLY CONTAMINATED ARTICLES AND BEFORE TAKING CARE OF ANOTHER PATIENT, HANDS SHOULD BE WASHED.**
- **ARTICLES** contaminated with infective material must be discarded or decontaminated.
- **AMBULANCE** - any surfaces contaminated with infective material must be disinfected.

DISEASES REQUIRING DRAINAGE/SECRETION PRECAUTIONS

DISEASES	INFECTIVE MATERIAL
Abscess, minor or limited	Pus
Burn infections, minor or limited	Pus
Conjunctivitis (except newborn)	Pus
Decubitus ulcer, infected, minor or limited	Pus
Skin infection, minor or limited	Pus
Wound infection, minor or limited	Pus
Anthrax	
Cutaneous	Pus
Inhalation	Respiratory secretions
Cellulitis, limited or minor	Pus

DISEASES	INFECTIVE MATERIAL
Closed cavity infections, minor or limited drainage	Pus
Clostridium Perfringens Gas gangrene	Pus
Cytomegalovirus	Pus
Endometritis - other than Group A strep	Vaginal Discharge
Furunculosis, Staph, not newborn	Pus
Gangrene; gas gangrene of wounds	Pus
Herpes Simplex, (fever blisters) mucocutaneous, recurrent	Lesion secretions
Herpes Zoster (Shingles), localized in non-compromised patient	Lesion secretions
Keratoconjunctivitis, infective	Purulent exudate
Mycobacteria, nontuberculosis, wound	Drainage
Bubonic Plague	Pus, drainage from lesions
Pneumonia, chlamydia	Respiratory secretions
Staphylococcal, skin, wound or burn, minor	Pus
Streptococcal (Group A) Skin, wound, or burn infection, minor	Pus
Pharyngitis	Respiratory secretions
Scarlet Fever	Respiratory secretions
Toxic Shock Syndrome	Vaginal discharge or Pus
Trachoma, acute	Purulent exudate
Tuberculosis, Extrapulmonary, draining lesion	Pus
Tularemia, draining lesion	Pus
Zoster (Varicella-Zoster) localized in non-compromised patient	Lesion secretions

General Isolation Guidelines

ENTERIC PRECAUTIONS

- **MASKS** are not indicated.
- **OUTERWEAR** must be worn by all persons who may be in contact with infective material.
- **GLOVES** must be worn by all persons who may be in contact with infective material or items contaminated with infective material.
- **HANDS MUST BE WASHED AFTER REMOVING PPE, AFTER TOUCHING THE PATIENT OR POTENTIALLY CONTAMINATED ARTICLES AND BEFORE TAKING CARE OF ANOTHER PATIENT.**
- **ARTICLES** contaminated with infective material must be discarded or decontaminated. All linens should be considered contaminated.
- **AMBULANCE** - any surfaces contaminated with infective material must be disinfected.

DISEASES REQUIRING ENTERIC PRECAUTIONS

DISEASES	INFECTIVE MATERIAL
Amebic Dysentery	Feces
Cholera	Feces
Coxsackievirus Disease	Feces & Respiratory secretions
Diarrhea	Feces
Echovirus	Feces & Respiratory secretions
Encephalitis	Feces
Entercolitis caused by **Clostridium difficile** or **Staph Aureus**	Feces
Enteroviral infection	Feces
Gastroenteritis caused by:	
Campylobacter	Feces
Cryptosporidium	Feces
Dientamoeba fragilis	Feces
Escherichia coli (E-coli)	Feces

DISEASES	INFECTIVE MATERIAL
Gastroenteritis caused by: *(Continued)*	
Giardia lamblia	Feces
Norwalk agent	Feces
Salmonella	Feces
Shigella	Feces
Vibrio parahaemolyticus	Feces
Viruses (Norwalk agent & rotavirus)	Feces
Yersinia enterocolitica	Feces
Unknown etiology	Feces
Hand, foot and mouth disease	Feces
Hepatitis, viral Type A and E	Feces
Herpangina	Feces
Meningitis, viral	Feces
Necrotizing Enterocolitis	Feces
Pleurodynia	Feces
Poliomyelitis	Feces
Typhoid Fever	Feces
Viral pericarditis, myocarditis, meningitis	Feces & Respiratory secretions

Symptom Specific Isolation Guidelines

In this section, you will find guidelines to be followed when caring for or transporting patients with unknown diagnoses, but who are displaying signs or symptoms suggestive of infectious diseases. It is recommended that each provider spend sufficient time to become familiar with the guidelines in this section, as you will most frequently be dealing with an unknown quantity rather than a named disease. Unfortunately, we can all remember those experiences where the patients we've transported were identified later as having an infectious disease.

KEY TO SYMBOLS

🖐 = Gloves   😷 = Mask & Goggle or Faceshield*   👕 = Gown/Outerwear   😷 = Mask

🆙 = Universal Precautions
  If possibility of contact with blood or body fluids = 🖐
  If possibility of spraying or splashing of blood = 🖐 😷 👕

🙂 = No special precautions, general good hygiene and principles of Universal Precautions

* 🕶 + 😷 = 😷 or 🙂

Symptom Specific Isolation Precautions

Precautions to be taken with patients suspected of infectious diseases based on symptoms.

SYMPTOMS	PRECAUTIONS	ISOLATION CATEGORY
BLOOD/BODY FLUIDS	UP	Blood/Body Fluids
COLD SORES	👋 👕	Drainage/Secretions
DIARRHEA	👋 👕	Enteric
DRAINING WOUNDS	👋 👕	Drainage/Secretions
FEVER		
■ without other symptoms		
Adults	😷(mask)	Respiratory
Infant/Child	👋 😷 👕 😷	Strict
■ with respiratory symptoms		
Adults	👋 👕	Drainage/Secretions
Infant/Child	👋 😷 👕 😷	Strict
■ with GI symptoms		
Adults	👋 👕	Enteric
Infant/Child	👋 👕	Enteric
■ with neurological symptoms		
Adults	👋 👕	Drainage/Secretions
Infant/Child	😷	Respiratory
■ with draining wound		
All	👋 👕	Drainage/Secretions

KEY TO SYMBOLS

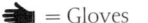 = Gloves   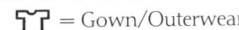 = Mask & Goggle or Faceshield   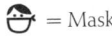 = Gown/Outerwear   = Mask

UP = Universal Precautions
   If possibility of contact with blood or body fluids =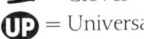
   If possibility of spraying or splashing of blood =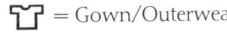

= No special precautions, general good hygiene and principles of Universal Precautions

SYMPTOMS	PRECAUTIONS	ISOLATION CATEGORY
JAUNDICE		
■ with history of liver or gallbladder disease	😊	NONE
■ without history of liver or gallbladder disease	UP	Blood & Body Fluids
PINK EYE		
■ conjunctivitis, draining or matted eyes	🖐 👕	Drainage/Secretions
RASHES AND/OR DRAINING RASHES		
■ with history of allergies	😊	NONE
■ without history of allergies or exposure to allergen	🖐 😷 👕 😷	Strict
RESPIRATORY SYMPTOMS		
■ with history or symptoms of chronic lung or heart problems	😊	NONE
■ with fever		
Adults	🖐 👕	Drainage/Secretions
Infant/Child	🖐 😷 👕 😷	Strict
■ without chronic history and with productive cough, weight loss, hemoptysis	😷	Respiratory
VOMITING		
■ with fever	🖐 👕	Drainage/Secretions
■ without fever	😊	NONE

KEY TO SYMBOLS

🖐 = Gloves   😷 = Mask & Goggle or Faceshield   👕 = Gown/Outerwear   😷 = Mask

UP = Universal Precautions
   If possibility of contact with blood or body fluids = 🖐
   If possibility of spraying or splashing of blood = 🖐 😷 👕

😊 = No special precautions, general good hygiene and principles of Universal Precautions

General Isolation Guidelines

DISEASE SPECIFIC ISOLATION GUIDLINES

What follows is an alphabetical listing of most of the infectious diseases a prehospital care provider might encounter. Included in this section is a quick reference chart describing the types of precautions to be used by the rescuer (mask, gloves, eye protection, outerwear protection) as well as the Isolation Category under which the disease is classified. This will permit cross referencing and allow the reader to identify not only the initial precautions to be taken, but also, by determining the Category of Isolation, they will be able to look back into that section and determine the infective material and what, if any, additional precautions need be taken.

KEY TO SYMBOLS

👆 = Gloves   😷 = Mask & Goggle or Faceshield*   👕 = Gown/Outerwear   😷 = Mask

UP = Universal Precautions
  If possibility of contact with blood or body fluids = 👆
  If possibility of spraying or splashing of blood = 👆 😷 👕

👤 = No special precautions, general good hygiene and principles of Universal Precautions

* 🕶️ + 😷 = 😷 or 🛡️

General Isolation Guidelines

DISEASE SPECIFIC ISOLATION PRECAUTIONS

DISEASE	PRECAUTIONS	ISOLATION CATEGORY
ABSCESS,		
■ etiology unknown		
Draining, major	🖐 😷 👕	STRICT
Draining, minor or limited	🖐 👕	DRAINAGE/ SECRETIONS
Not draining	🙂	NONE
ACQUIRED IMMUNO-DEFICIENCY SYNDROME (AIDS)	UP	BLOOD/BODY FLUIDS
ACTINOMYCOSIS,		
■ all lesions	🙂	NONE
ADENOVIRUS,		
■ respiratory in		
Infants & Children	🖐 😷 👕 😷	STRICT
AMEBIASIS		
■ Dysentery	🖐 👕	ENTERIC
■ Liver Abscess	🙂	NONE
ANTHRAX		
■ Cutaneous	🖐 👕	DRAINAGE/ SECRETIONS
■ Inhalation	🖐 👕	DRAINAGE/ SECRETIONS

KEY TO SYMBOLS

🖐 = Gloves   😷 = Mask & Goggle or Faceshield   👕 = Gown/Outerwear   😷 = Mask

UP = Universal Precautions
    If possibility of contact with blood or body fluids = 🖐
    If possibility of spraying or splashing of blood = 🖐 😷 👕

🙂 = No special precautions, general good hygiene and principles of Universal Precautions

General Isolation Guidelines

DISEASE	PRECAUTIONS	ISOLATION CATEGORY
ARTHROPODBORNE VIRAL ENCEPHALITIDES ■ (eastern equine, western equine, and Venezuelan equine encephalomyelitis, St. Louis and California encephalitis)	UP	BLOOD/BODY FLUIDS
ARTHROPODBORNE VIRAL FEVERS ■ (dengue, yellow fever and Colorado tick fever)	UP	BLOOD/BODY FLUIDS
ASCARIASIS	☻	NONE
BABESIOSIS	UP	BLOOD/BODY FLUIDS
BLASTOMYCOSIS, ■ North American, cutanenous or pulmonary	☻	NONE
BOTULISM	☻	NONE
BRONCHIOLITIS, ■ etiology unknown,		
Infants & young children	🖐 😷 👕 😷	STRICT
BRONCHITIS, ■ etiology unknown,		
Adult	☻	NONE
Infants & children	🖐 😷 👕 😷	STRICT

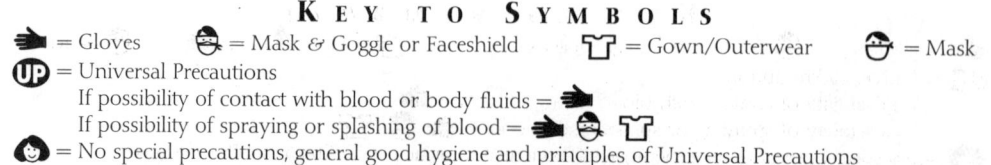

KEY TO SYMBOLS
🖐 = Gloves   😷 = Mask & Goggle or Faceshield   👕 = Gown/Outerwear   😷 = Mask
UP = Universal Precautions
   If possibility of contact with blood or body fluids = 🖐
   If possibility of spraying or splashing of blood = 🖐 😷 👕
☻ = No special precautions, general good hygiene and principles of Universal Precautions

General Isolation Guidelines

DISEASE	PRECAUTIONS	ISOLATION CATEGORY
BRUCELLOSIS ■ (undulant fever, Malta fever, Mediterranean fever) Draining lesions, limited or minor	UP	BLOOD/BODY FLUIDS
BURN WOUND ■ major, draining	Gloves, Mask & Goggle, Gown	STRICT
■ limited or minor	Gloves, Gown	DRAINAGE/ SECRETIONS
CAMPYLOBACTER ■ gastroenteritis	Gloves, Gown	ENTERIC
CANDIDIASIS, ■ all forms including moniliasis, thrush	No special precautions	NONE
CAT–SCRATCH FEVER	No special precautions	NONE
CELLULITIS ■ Draining, limited or minor	Gloves, Gown	DRAINAGE/ SECRETIONS
■ Intact skin	No special precautions	NONE
CHANCROID (soft chancre)	No special precautions	NONE
CHICKENPOX (varicella)	Gloves, Mask & Goggle, Gown, Mask	STRICT

KEY TO SYMBOLS

- 👉 = Gloves
- 😷 = Mask & Goggle or Faceshield
- 👕 = Gown/Outerwear
- 😷 = Mask
- UP = Universal Precautions
    - If possibility of contact with blood or body fluids = 👉
    - If possibility of spraying or splashing of blood = 👉 😷 👕
- 🙂 = No special precautions, general good hygiene and principles of Universal Precautions

DISEASE	PRECAUTIONS			ISOLATION CATEGORY
CHLAMYDIA trachomatis infection				
■ Conjunctivitis	Gloves	Gown		DRAINAGE/SECRETIONS
■ Genital	Gloves	Gown		DRAINAGE/SECRETIONS
■ Respiratory	Gloves	Gown		DRAINAGE/SECRETIONS
CHOLERA	Gloves	Gown		ENTERIC
CLOSED-CAVITY INFECTION				
■ Draining, limited or minor	Gloves	Gown		DRAINAGE/SECRETIONS
■ Not draining	No special			NONE
CLOSTRIDIUM PERFRINGENS				
■ Food poisoning	No special			NONE
■ Gas Gangrene	Gloves	Gown		DRAINAGE/SECRETIONS
■ Other	No special			NONE
COCCIDIOMYCOSIS				
■ Draining lesions	No special			NONE
■ Pneumonia	No special			NONE
COLORADO TICK FEVER	Universal Precautions			BLOOD/BODY FLUIDS
COMMON COLD				
■ Adults	No special			NONE
■ Infants & young children	Gloves	Mask	Gown	STRICT

Key to Symbols

- 🖐 = Gloves
- 😷 = Mask & Goggle or Faceshield
- 👕 = Gown/Outerwear
- 🎭 = Mask
- **UP** = Universal Precautions
    - If possibility of contact with blood or body fluids = 🖐
    - If possibility of spraying or splashing of blood = 🖐 😷 👕
- 👩 = No special precautions, general good hygiene and principles of Universal Precautions

General Isolation Guidelines

DISEASE	PRECAUTIONS	ISOLATION CATEGORY
CONGENITAL RUBELLA	Gloves, Mask & Goggle, Gown, Mask	STRICT
CONJUNCTIVITIS,		
■ acute bacterial (sore eye, pink eye)	Gloves, Gown	DRAINAGE/SECRETIONS
■ Chlamydia	Gloves, Gown	DRAINAGE/SECRETIONS
■ Gonococcal		
Adult	Gloves, Gown	DRAINAGE/SECRETIONS
Newborns	Gloves, Mask & Goggle, Gown, Mask	STRICT
■ Viral	Gloves, Gown	DRAINAGE/SECRETIONS
■ Unknown etiology	Gloves, Gown	DRAINAGE/SECRETIONS
CORONAVIRUS INFECTION		
■ respiratory		
Adult	No special precautions	NONE
Infants & young children	Gloves, Mask & Goggle, Gown, Mask	STRICT
COXSACKIEVIRUS DISEASE	Gloves, Gown	ENTERIC
CREUTZFELDT–JAKOB DISEASE	Universal Precautions	BLOOD/BODY FLUIDS
CROUP	Gloves, Mask & Goggle, Gown, Mask	STRICT
CRYPTOCOCCOSIS	No special precautions	NONE
CYSTICERCOSIS	No special precautions	NONE

KEY TO SYMBOLS

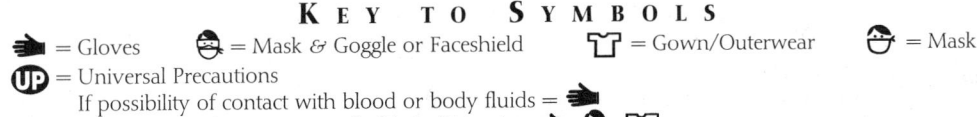

- = Gloves
- = Mask & Goggle or Faceshield
- = Gown/Outerwear
- = Mask
- **UP** = Universal Precautions
  - If possibility of contact with blood or body fluids = Gloves
  - If possibility of spraying or splashing of blood = Gloves, Mask & Goggle, Gown
- = No special precautions, general good hygiene and principles of Universal Precautions

DISEASE	PRECAUTIONS	ISOLATION CATEGORY
CYTOMEGALOVIRUS	Gloves, Gown	DRAINAGE/SECRETIONS
DECUBITUS ULCER, ■ infected		
Draining, major	Gloves, Mask & Goggle, Gown	STRICT
Draining, minor	Gloves, Gown	DRAINAGE/SECRETIONS
DENGUE	UP	BLOOD/BODY FLUIDS
DIARRHEA, ■ acute	Gloves, Gown	ENTERIC
DIPHTHERIA		
■ Cutaneous	Gloves, Mask & Goggle, Gown, Mask	STRICT
■ Pharyngeal	Gloves, Mask & Goggle, Gown, Mask	STRICT
ECHINOCOCCOSIS	No special precautions	NONE
ECHOVIRUS DISEASE	Gloves, Gown	ENTERIC
ECZEMA VACCINATION ■ vaccinia	Gloves, Mask & Goggle, Gown, Mask	STRICT
ENCEPHALITIS ■ or encephalomyelitis, etiology unknown	Gloves, Gown	ENTERIC

KEY TO SYMBOLS

- = Gloves
- = Mask & Goggle or Faceshield
- = Gown/Outerwear
- = Mask
- **UP** = Universal Precautions
  - If possibility of contact with blood or body fluids = Gloves
  - If possibility of spraying or splashing of blood = Gloves, Mask & Goggle, Gown
- = No special precautions, general good hygiene and principles of Universal Precautions

General Isolation Guidelines

DISEASE	PRECAUTIONS	ISOLATION CATEGORY
ENDOMETRITIS		
■ Group A Strep	Gloves, Mask & Goggle, Gown, Mask	STRICT
■ Other	Gloves, Gown	DRAINAGE/SECRETIONS
ENTEROBIASIS		
■ (pinworms)	No special precautions	NONE
ENTEROCOLITIS		
■ Clostridium difficile	Gloves, Gown	ENTERIC
■ Staphylococcus	Gloves, Gown	ENTERIC
ENTEROVIRAL INFECTION	Gloves, Gown	ENTERIC
EPIGLOTTITIS (H.Flu)	Mask & Goggle	RESPIRATORY
EPSTEIN-BARR VIRUS INFECTION, ■ including mononucleosis	Gloves, Gown	DRAINAGE/SECRETIONS
ERYSIPELOID	No special precautions	NONE
ERYTHEMA INFECTIOSUM	Mask & Goggle	RESPIRATORY
ESCHERICHIA COLI ■ gastroenteritis	Gloves, Gown	ENTERIC
FEVER OF UNKNOWN ORIGIN ■ (FUO)		
Adults	Mask & Goggle, Mask	RESPIRATORY
Infants & children	Gloves, Mask & Goggle, Gown, Mask	STRICT

KEY TO SYMBOLS

- = Gloves
- = Mask & Goggle or Faceshield
- = Gown/Outerwear
- = Mask
- **UP** = Universal Precautions
  - If possibility of contact with blood or body fluids = Gloves
  - If possibility of spraying or splashing of blood = Gloves, Mask & Goggle, Gown
- = No special precautions, general good hygiene and principles of Universal Precautions

DISEASE	PRECAUTIONS	ISOLATION CATEGORY
FOOD POISONING		
■ Botulism	😀	NONE
■ Clostridium perfringen or welchii	😀	NONE
■ Salmonellosis	🖐 👕	ENTERIC
■ Staphylococcal	😀	NONE
FURUNCULOSIS, ■ staph		
Adults	🖐 👕	DRAINAGE/ SECRETIONS
Infants & children	🖐 😷 👕	STRICT
GANGRENE, Gas	🖐 👕	DRAINAGE SECRETIONS
GASTROENTERITIS		
■ Campylobacter	🖐 👕	ENTERIC
■ Clostridium difficile	🖐 👕	ENTERIC
■ Cryptosporidium	🖐 👕	ENTERIC
■ Dientamoeba fragilis	🖐 👕	ENTERIC
■ Escherichia coli	🖐 👕	ENTERIC
■ Giardia lamblia	🖐 👕	ENTERIC
■ Rotavirus	🖐 👕	ENTERIC
■ Salmonella	🖐 👕	ENTERIC
■ Shigella	🖐 👕	ENTERIC

KEY TO SYMBOLS

🖐 = Gloves   😷 = Mask & Goggle or Faceshield   👕 = Gown/Outerwear   😷 = Mask

UP = Universal Precautions
    If possibility of contact with blood or body fluids = 🖐
    If possibility of spraying or splashing of blood = 🖐 😷 👕

😀 = No special precautions, general good hygiene and principles of Universal Precautions

General Isolation Guidelines

DISEASE	PRECAUTIONS	ISOLATION CATEGORY
GASTROENTERITIS *(Continued)*		
■ Unknown etiology	👋 👕	ENTERIC
■ Vibrio parahaemolyticus	👋 👕	ENTERIC
■ Viral	👋 👕	ENTERIC
■ Yersinia enterocolitica	👋 👕	ENTERIC
GERMAN MEASLES (rubella)	👋 😷 👕 😷	STRICT
GIARDIASIS	👋 👕	ENTERIC
GONOCOCCAL OPHTHALMIA NEONATORUM	👋 😷 👕	STRICT
GONORRHEA	👩	NONE
GRANULOCYTOPENIA	👩	NONE
GRANULOMA INGUINALE	👩	NONE
GUILLAIN–BARRE SYNDROME	👩	NONE
HAND, FOOT, AND MOUTH DISEASE	👋 👕	ENTERIC
HEMORRHAGIC FEVERS ■ (i.e.) Lassa fever	👋 😷 👕 😷	STRICT
HEPATITIS, VIRAL		
■ Type A	👋 👕	ENTERIC
■ Type B	UP	BLOOD/BODY FLUIDS

KEY TO SYMBOLS

👋 = Gloves　　😷 = Mask & Goggle or Faceshield　　👕 = Gown/Outerwear　　😷 = Mask

UP = Universal Precautions
　　If possibility of contact with blood or body fluids = 👋
　　If possibility of spraying or splashing of blood = 👋 😷 👕

👩 = No special precautions, general good hygiene and principles of Universal Precautions

DISEASE	PRECAUTIONS	ISOLATION CATEGORY
HEPATITIS, VIRAL (Continued)		
■ Type C	UP	BLOOD/BODY FLUIDS
■ Delta Hepatitis	UP	BLOOD/BODY FLUIDS
■ Type E	Gloves, Gown	ENTERIC
■ Non-A, Non-B	UP	BLOOD/BODY FLUIDS
■ Unspecified	UP	BLOOD/BODY FLUIDS
HERPANGINA	Gloves, Gown	ENTERIC
HERPES SIMPLEX		
■ Encephalitis	No special precautions	NONE
■ Mucocutaneous, disseminated or primary, severe	Gloves, Mask & Goggle, Gown, Mask	STRICT
■ Mucocutaneous, recurrent	Gloves, Gown	DRAINAGE/ SECRETIONS
■ Neonatal	Gloves, Mask & Goggle, Gown, Mask	STRICT
HERPES ZOSTER (varicella)		
■ Localized in immunocompromised patient or disseminated	Gloves, Mask & Goggle, Gown, Mask	STRICT
■ Localized in normal patient	Gloves, Gown	DRAINAGE/ SECRETIONS

KEY TO SYMBOLS

- = Gloves
- = Mask & Goggle or Faceshield
- = Gown/Outerwear
- = Mask
- **UP** = Universal Precautions
  - If possibility of contact with blood or body fluids = Gloves
  - If possibility of spraying or splashing of blood = Gloves, Mask & Goggle, Gown
- = No special precautions, general good hygiene and principles of Universal Precautions

General Isolation Guidelines

DISEASE	PRECAUTIONS	ISOLATION CATEGORY
HISTOPLASMOSIS	🙂	NONE
HOOKWORM DISEASE	🙂	NONE
HUMAN IMMUNO-DEFICIENCY VIRUS (HIV)	UP	BLOOD/BODY FLUIDS
IMMUNOCOMPROMISED STATUS	🙂	NONE
IMPETIGO	🖐 😷 👕	STRICT
INFECTIOUS MONONUCLEOSIS	🖐 👕	DRAINAGE/SECRETIONS
INFLUENZA ■ Adults	🙂	NONE
■ Infants & children	🖐 😷 👕 🎭	STRICT
CREUTZFELDT-JAKOB DISEASE	UP	BLOOD/BODY FLUIDS
KAWASAKI SYNDROME	🙂	NONE
KERATOCONJUNCTIVITIS, ■ infective	🖐 👕	DRAINAGE/SECRETIONS
LASSA FEVER	🖐 😷 👕 🎭	STRICT
LEGIONNAIRES' DISEASE	🙂	NONE
LEPROSY	🙂	NONE
LEPTOSPIROSIS	UP	BLOOD/BODY FLUIDS

KEY TO SYMBOLS

🖐 = Gloves   😷 = Mask & Goggle or Faceshield   👕 = Gown/Outerwear   🎭 = Mask

UP = Universal Precautions
  If possibility of contact with blood or body fluids = 🖐
  If possibility of spraying or splashing of blood = 🖐 😷 👕

🙂 = No special precautions, general good hygiene and principles of Universal Precautions

DISEASE	PRECAUTIONS	ISOLATION CATEGORY
LISTERIOSIS	🙂	NONE
LYME DISEASE	🙂	NONE
LYMPHOCYTIC ■ choriomeningitis	🙂	NONE
LYMPHOGRANULOMA ■ venereum	🙂	NONE
MALARIA	UP	BLOOD/BODY FLUIDS
MARBURG VIRUS DISEASE	👉 😷 👕 😷	STRICT
MEASLES (rubeola)	😷	RESPIRATORY
MELIOIDOSIS	🙂	NONE
MENINGITIS ■ Aseptic	👉 😷 👕 😷	STRICT
■ Bacterial, gram-negative enteric, in neonates	🙂	NONE
■ Fungal	🙂	NONE
■ Haemophilus influenzae (H.flu), known or suspected	😷	RESPIRATORY
■ Listeria monocytogenes	🙂	NONE
■ Neisseria meningitidis (meningococcal, known or suspected)	😷	RESPIRATORY

Key to Symbols

👉 = Gloves   😷 = Mask & Goggle or Faceshield   👕 = Gown/Outerwear   😷 = Mask

UP = Universal Precautions
  If possibility of contact with blood or body fluids = 👉
  If possibility of spraying or splashing of blood = 👉 😷 👕

🙂 = No special precautions, general good hygiene and principles of Universal Precautions

General Isolation Guidelines

DISEASE	PRECAUTIONS	ISOLATION CATEGORY
MENINGITIS *(Continued)*		
■ Pneumococcal	🙂	NONE
■ Tuberculosis	🙂	NONE
■ Other bacterial	🙂	NONE
MENINGOCOCCAL PNEUMONIA	😷	RESPIRATORY
MENINGOCOCCEMIA ■ (meningococcal sepsis)	😷	RESPIRATORY
MOLLUSCUM CONTAGIOSUM	🙂	NONE
MUCORMYCOSIS	🙂	NONE
MULTIPLY-RESISTANT ORGANISMS, INFECTION OR COLONIZATION		
■ Gastrointestinal	🖐 😷 👕	STRICT
■ Respiratory	🖐 😷 👕	STRICT
■ Skin, wound, or burn	🖐 😷 👕	STRICT
■ Urinary	🖐 😷 👕	STRICT
MUMPS	😷	RESPIRATORY
MYCOBACTERIA, nontuberculous (atypical)		
■ Pulmonary	🙂	NONE
■ Wound	🖐 👕	DRAINAGE/SECRETIONS
MYCOPLASMA PNEUMONIA	🙂	NONE

KEY TO SYMBOLS

🖐 = Gloves   😷 = Mask & Goggle or Faceshield   👕 = Gown/Outerwear   😷 = Mask

UP = Universal Precautions
  If possibility of contact with blood or body fluids = 🖐
  If possibility of spraying or splashing of blood = 🖐 😷 👕

🙂 = No special precautions, general good hygiene and principles of Universal Precautions

DISEASE	PRECAUTIONS	ISOLATION CATEGORY
NECROTIZING ENTERCOLITIS	gloves, gown	ENTERIC
NEUTROPENIA	none	NONE
NOCARDIOSIS		
■ Draining lesions	none	NONE
■ Other	none	NONE
NORWALK AGENT		
■ gastroenteritis	gloves, gown	ENTERIC
ORF	none	NONE
PARAINFLUENZA VIRUS INFECTION in		
■ Infants & young children	gloves, mask & goggle, gown, mask	STRICT
PEDICULOSIS	gloves, mask & goggle, gown	STRICT
PERTUSSIS		
■ (whooping cough)	mask	RESPIRATORY
PHARYNGITIS, INFECTIVE,		
■ etiology unknown		
Adults	none	NONE
Infants & children	gloves, mask & goggle, gown, mask	STRICT
PINWORM INFECTION	none	NONE
PLAGUE		
■ Bubonic	gloves, gown	DRAINAGE/ SECRETIONS
■ Pneumonic	gloves, mask & goggle, gown, mask	STRICT

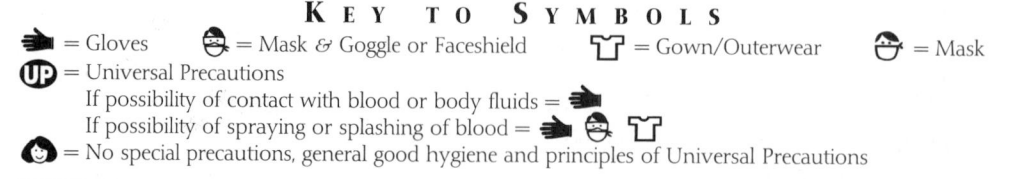

KEY TO SYMBOLS

🖐 = Gloves   😷 = Mask & Goggle or Faceshield   👕 = Gown/Outerwear   😷 = Mask

UP = Universal Precautions
  If possibility of contact with blood or body fluids = 🖐
  If possibility of spraying or splashing of blood = 🖐 😷 👕

👩 = No special precautions, general good hygiene and principles of Universal Precautions

General Isolation Guidelines

DISEASE	PRECAUTIONS	ISOLATION CATEGORY
PLEURODYNIA	Gloves, Gown	ENTERIC
PNEUMONIA		
■ Bacterial not listed elsewhere	None	NONE
■ Chlamydia	Gloves, Gown	DRAINAGE/SECRETIONS
■ Etiology unknown		
Adults	Gloves, Gown	DRAINAGE/SECRETIONS
Infants & children	Gloves, Mask&Goggle, Gown, Mask	STRICT
■ Fungal	None	NONE
■ Haemophilus influenzae		
Adults	None	NONE
Infants & children	Mask	RESPIRATORY
■ Legionnella	None	NONE
■ Meningococcal	Mask	RESPIRATORY
■ Multiply-resistant bacterial	Gloves, Mask, Gown	STRICT
■ Mycoplasma	None	NONE
■ Pneumococcal	None	NONE
■ Pneumocystis carinii	None	NONE
■ Staphylococcus Aureus	Gloves, Mask&Goggle, Gown, Mask	STRICT
■ Steptococcus group A	Gloves, Mask&Goggle, Gown, Mask	STRICT

Key to Symbols

- = Gloves
- = Mask & Goggle or Faceshield
- = Gown/Outerwear
- = Mask
- **UP** = Universal Precautions
  - If possibility of contact with blood or body fluids = Gloves
  - If possibility of spraying or splashing of blood = Gloves, Mask&Goggle, Gown
- = No special precautions, general good hygiene and principles of Universal Precautions

DISEASE	PRECAUTIONS	ISOLATION CATEGORY
PNEUMONIA (Continued) ■ Viral		
Adults	😊	NONE
Infants & children	🧤 😷 👕 😷	STRICT
POLIOMYELITIS	🧤 👕	ENTERIC
PSITTACOSIS	😊	NONE
Q FEVER	😊	NONE
RABIES	🧤 😷 👕 😷	STRICT
RAT-BITE FEVER	UP	BLOOD/BODY FLUIDS
RELAPSING FEVER	UP	BLOOD/BODY FLUIDS
RESISTANT BACTERIAL ■ (see multiply-resistant bacteria)		
RESPIRATORY INFECTIOUS DISEASE ■ acute (if not covered elsewhere)		
Adults	😊	NONE
Infants & young children	🧤 😷 👕 😷	STRICT
RESPIRATORY SYNCYTIAL VIRUS ■ (RSV) in		
Infants & young children	🧤 😷 👕 😷	STRICT

KEY TO SYMBOLS

🧤 = Gloves   😷 = Mask & Goggle or Faceshield   👕 = Gown/Outerwear   😷 = Mask

UP = Universal Precautions
    If possibility of contact with blood or body fluids = 🧤
    If possibility of spraying or splashing of blood = 🧤 😷 👕

😊 = No special precautions, general good hygiene and principles of Universal Precautions

General Isolation Guidelines

DISEASE	PRECAUTIONS	ISOLATION CATEGORY
REYE'S SYNDROME	😊	NONE
RHEUMATIC FEVER	😊	NONE
RHINOVIRUS INFECTION, ■ respiratory		
Adults	😊	NONE
Infants & young children	👋 😷 👕 🎭	STRICT
RICKETTSIAL FEVERS, ■ tick-borne (Rocky Mountain spotted fever, tickborne typhus fever)	UP	BLOOD/BODY FLUIDS
RICKETTSIALPOX	😊	NONE
RINGWORM	😊	NONE
RITTER'S DISEASE (Scalded Skin Syndrome)	👋 😷 👕	STRICT
ROCKY MOUNTAIN SPOTTED FEVER	UP	BLOOD/BODY FLUIDS
ROSEOLA INFANTUM	😊	NONE
ROTAVIRUS INFECTION ■ viral gastroenteritis	👋 👕	ENTERIC
RUBELLA (German Measles)	👋 😷 👕 🎭	STRICT
SALMONELLOSIS	👋 👕	ENTERIC

KEY TO SYMBOLS

👋 = Gloves   😷 = Mask & Goggle or Faceshield   👕 = Gown/Outerwear   🎭 = Mask

UP = Universal Precautions
    If possibility of contact with blood or body fluids = 👋
    If possibility of spraying or splashing of blood = 👋 😷 👕

😊 = No special precautions, general good hygiene and principles of Universal Precautions

DISEASE	PRECAUTIONS	ISOLATION CATEGORY
SCABIES	Gloves, Gown	STRICT
SCALDED SKIN SYNDROME, ■ staph, (Ritter's disease)	Gloves, Mask & Goggle, Gown	STRICT
SCHISTOSOMIASIS	No special precautions	NONE
SHIGELLOSIS	Gloves, Gown	ENTERIC
SMALLPOX	Gloves, Mask & Goggle, Gown, Mask	STRICT
SPOROTRICHOSIS	No special precautions	NONE
SPIRILLIUM MINUS DISEASE	Universal Precautions	BLOOD/BODY FLUIDS
STAPHYLOCOCCAL DISEASE (S. aureus) ■ Skin wound, or burn infection		
Major	Gloves, Mask & Goggle, Gown	STRICT
Minor or limited	Gloves, Gown	DRAINAGE/SECRETIONS
■ Enterocolitis	Gloves, Gown	ENTERIC
■ Pneumonia or draining lung abscess	Gloves, Mask & Goggle, Gown	STRICT
■ Scalded skin syndrome	Gloves, Mask & Goggle, Gown	STRICT
■ Toxic shock syndrome	Gloves, Gown	DRAINAGE/SECRETIONS

KEY TO SYMBOLS

- 🖐 = Gloves
- 😷 = Mask & Goggle or Faceshield
- 👕 = Gown/Outerwear
- 🎭 = Mask
- **UP** = Universal Precautions
  - If possibility of contact with blood or body fluids = 🖐
  - If possibility of spraying or splashing of blood = 🖐 😷 👕
- 👩 = No special precautions, general good hygiene and principles of Universal Precautions

General Isolation Guidelines

DISEASE	PRECAUTIONS	ISOLATION CATEGORY
STREPTOBACILLUS ■ moniliformis	UP	BLOOD/BODY FLUIDS
STREPTOCOCCAL DISEASE (group A) ■ Skin, wound, or burn infection		
Major	Gloves, Mask & Goggle, Gown	STRICT
Minor or limited	Gloves, Gown	DRAINAGE/SECRETIONS
■ Endometritis	Gloves, Mask & Goggle, Gown	STRICT
■ Pharyngitis	Gloves, Gown	DRAINAGE/SECRETIONS
■ Pneumonia	Gloves, Mask & Goggle, Gown	STRICT
■ Scarlet fever	Gloves, Gown	DRAINAGE/SECRETIONS
STREPTOCOCCAL DISEASE (group B) ■ Neonatal	No special precautions	NONE
STREPTOCOCCAL DISEASE ■ not group A or B	No special precautions	NONE
STRONGYLOIDIASIS	No special precautions	NONE

KEY TO SYMBOLS

- 🖐 = Gloves
- 😷 = Mask & Goggle or Faceshield
- 👕 = Gown/Outerwear
- 🎭 = Mask
- UP = Universal Precautions
  - If possibility of contact with blood or body fluids = 🖐
  - If possibility of spraying or splashing of blood = 🖐 😷 👕
- 👩 = No special precautions, general good hygiene and principles of Universal Precautions

DISEASE	PRECAUTIONS	ISOLATION CATEGORY
SYPHILIS		
■ Skin and mucous membrane, including	Gloves, Gown	DRAINAGE/ SECRETIONS &
■ congenital, primary and secondary	Universal Precautions	BLOOD/BODY FLUIDS
■ Latent (tertiary) & seropositivity without lesions	No special precautions	NONE
TAPEWORM DISEASE		
■ Hymenolepis nana	No special precautions	NONE
■ Taenia solium (pork)	No special precautions	NONE
TETANUS	No special precautions	NONE
TINEA		
■ (fungus infection dermatophytosis, dermatomycosis, ringworm)	No special precautions	NONE
TOXOPLASMOSIS	No special precautions	NONE
TOXIC SHOCK SYNDROME		
■ (staph disease)	Gloves, Gown	DRAINAGE/ SECRETIONS
TRACHOMA, acute	Gloves, Gown	DRAINAGE/ SECRETIONS
TRENCH MOUTH		
■ (Vincent's angina)	No special precautions	NONE
TRICHINOSIS	No special precautions	NONE

KEY TO SYMBOLS

- = Gloves
- = Mask & Goggle or Faceshield
- = Gown/Outerwear
- = Mask
- **UP** = Universal Precautions
  - If possibility of contact with blood or body fluids = Gloves
  - If possibility of spraying or splashing of blood = Gloves, Mask & Goggle, Gown
- = No special precautions, general good hygiene and principles of Universal Precautions

General Isolation Guidelines

DISEASE	PRECAUTIONS	ISOLATION CATEGORY
TRICHOMONIASIS	😊	NONE
TRICHURIASIS ■ (whipworm disease)	😊	NONE
TUBERCULOSIS		
■ Extrapulmonary, draining lesion	🧤 👕	DRAINAGE/SECRETIONS
■ Meningitis	😊	NONE
■ Pulmonary confirmed or suspected active	😷	RESPIRATORY
■ Skin test positive with no evidence of current pulmonary disease	😊	NONE
TULAREMIA		
■ Draining lesion	🧤 👕	DRAINAGE/SECRETIONS
■ Pulmonary	😊	NONE
TYPHOID FEVER	🧤 👕	ENTERIC
TYPHUS	😊	NONE
URINARY TRACT INFECTION	😊	NONE
VACCINIA		
■ At vaccination site	🧤 👕	DRAINAGE/SECRETIONS
■ Generalized and progressisve eczema vaccinatum	🧤 😷 👕	STRICT

Key to Symbols

🧤 = Gloves 😷 = Mask & Goggle or Faceshield 👕 = Gown/Outerwear 😷 = Mask

UP = Universal Precautions
   If possibility of contact with blood or body fluids = 🧤
   If possibility of spraying or splashing of blood = 🧤 😷 👕

😊 = No special precautions, general good hygiene and principles of Universal Precautions

DISEASE	PRECAUTIONS	ISOLATION CATEGORY
VARICELLA (chickenpox)	👉 😷 👕 🎭	STRICT
VARIOLA (smallpox)	👉 😷 👕 🎭	STRICT
VIBRIO PARAHAEMOLYTICUS ■ gastroenteritis	👉 👕	ENTERIC
VINCENT'S ANGINA	🙂	NONE
VIRAL DISEASES ■ Pericarditis, myocarditis or meningitis	👉 👕	ENTERIC
■ Respiratory		
Adults	🙂	NONE
Infants & children	👉 😷 👕 🎭	STRICT
WHOOPING COUGH ■ (pertussis)	🎭	RESPIRATORY
WOUND INFECTIONS ■ Major	👉 😷 👕	STRICT
■ Minor or limited	👉 👕	DRAINAGE/ SECRETIONS
YAWS	👉 👕	DRAINAGE/ SECRETIONS
YELLOW FEVER	UP	BLOOD/BODY FLUIDS
YERSINIA ENTEROCOLITICA ■ gastroenteritis	👉 👕	ENTERIC

Key to Symbols

- 👉 = Gloves
- 😷 = Mask & Goggle or Faceshield
- 👕 = Gown/Outerwear
- 🎭 = Mask
- UP = Universal Precautions
  - If possibility of contact with blood or body fluids = 👉
  - If possibility of spraying or splashing of blood = 👉 😷 👕
- 🙂 = No special precautions, general good hygiene and principles of Universal Precautions

General Isolation Guidelines

DISEASE	PRECAUTIONS	ISOLATION CATEGORY
ZOSTER (varicella zoster)		
■ Localized in immunocompromised or disseminated	🖐 😷 👕 😷	STRICT
■ Localized in normal patient	🖐 😷 👕 😷	DRAINAGE/ SECRETIONS
ZYGOMYCOSIS		
■ (phycomycosis, mucormycosis)	👩	NONE

KEY TO SYMBOLS

🖐 = Gloves   😷 = Mask & Goggle or Faceshield   👕 = Gown/Outerwear   😷 = Mask

UP = Universal Precautions
  If possibility of contact with blood or body fluids = 🖐
  If possibility of spraying or splashing of blood = 🖐 😷 👕

👩 = No special precautions, general good hygiene and principles of Universal Precautions

Notes

General Isolation Guidelines

Preparing an Isolation Patient for Transport

A. Before entering room completely cover stretcher or wheelchair with a large clean sheet.

B. Drape the side of the stretcher that will be next to the bed with a clean draw sheet.

C. Personnel shall use appropriate gloves, face protection and outerwear protection as indicated by type of disease or symptoms.

D. Enter room and place patient on stretcher.

E. With the patient on the stretcher cover patient with the inside of the sheet, leaving clean side out, and bring sides of large sheet and blanket or cot cover up over the patient.

F. Use mask ON PATIENT if respiratory, strict, or protective isolation precautions are being utilized, provided patient will tolerate.

G. Cover patient with additional blankets or cot cover as necessary for patient comfort. Avoid contaminating these outer coverings.

H. To remove patient from stretcher, reverse the above order of events.

I. All contaminated linens should be disposed of in the patient's room if possible; or if not to be left at the hospital, they should be rolled so as to leave the clean side out and then disposed of in contaminated linen bag in vehicle and returned to station. Special precautions should be followed if linens have been contaminated by patient's blood or body fluids; see care of contaminated articles. For further guidelines refer to Disease or Symptoms Specific Charts.

Chapter Three

Employee Exposure & Illness

Guidelines for Employees Exposed to Infectious Diseases and with Known or Suspected Infectious Diseases

Notes

POLICY STATEMENT

When employees are exposed to infectious diseases, a supervisor should immediately be notified by the employee. An incident report describing the circumstances surrounding the suspected exposure incident should be completed. The supervisor will refer to this document for further action. In the event that prophylactic treatment or testing is needed, the supervisor will notify the employee and provide the employee with an authorization form for treatment. The employee will report with authorization form to _____ (hospital/clinic/physician) for appropriate treatment and consultation.

Employees having or being exposed to any of the diseases found in the following guidelines, should be tested/treated in accordance with these guidelines. Any deviations from treatment/testing shall be approved by the company/agency physician and management.

NOTE: Almost any transmissible infection may occur in the community at large and can affect both employee and patient. Only those diseases that occur frequently in the prehospital care setting or are most important to personnel are discussed in the following guidelines.

Approved this date_____

_____
Authorizing Signature

_____
Consulting Physician

Notes

BLOODEBORNE PATHOGENS

A. ACQUIRED IMMUNE DEFICIENCY SYNDROME (AIDS)

1. **Identification:** A viral disease transmitted through semen, blood and certain body fluids; can be transmitted through sexual intercourse, contaminated needles, transfusions, and to babies born to infected mothers.

    HIV1 and HIV2 are human retroviruses. Once inside the body, the virus begins to replicate in many cells of the body leading to opportunistic infections, neurologic disease and/or cancer.

    Infection with HIV can be identified in most, but not all patients, by testing the blood for presence of HIV antibodies. Usually the blood is tested using the ELISA technique. This test is very sensitive and economical. If the test is negative, no HIV antibodies are present. If the test is positive, a second ELISA test is run on the blood sample. If this second test is positive, a confirmatory test is conducted using the Western Blot technique. This test is more specific but less sensitive than the ELISA and is used to validate the first test. If both tests are positive, it is indicative of the presence of HIV antibodies and HIV infection. One major disadvantage to antibody testing is that if the individual being tested was recently infected and has not developed antibodies the test will be negative. This window period, when an individual is infected and capable of transmitting HIV virus to others but is antibody negative, may be as long as 6-12 months. In addition, patients with advanced HIV infection may be unable to make antibody any longer and they may, on occasion, have a negative test. Newer tests are currently being developed that will test for the presence of virus itself rather than antibodies, thus allowing for earlier detection of disease.

    AIDS is definded as the presence of an opportunistic infection or unusual cancer in a patient with no known cause of immunodeficiency other than HIV infection, or by the presence of HIV infection with severe depression of the immune system (defined as a CD4 count less than 200 cells/mm3 in persons over 13 years of age).

DISEASES ASSOCIATED WITH HIV/AIDS

- Parasitic diseases
  Toxoplasmosis
  Cryptosporidiosis

- Fungal diseases
  Candidiasis
  Pneumocystis carinii pneumonia
  Histoplasmosis
  Cryptococcosis

DISEASES ASSOCIATED WITH HIV/AIDS (Continued)

- Viral diseases
  Cytomegalovirus
  Herpes Simplex
  Varicella Zoster (chickenpox, shingles)

- Cancer/neoplastic diseases
  Kaposi's sarcoma
  Non-Hodgkin's Lymphoma
  Primary CNS Lymphoma
  Invasive cervical cancer

- Bacterial infections
  Mycobacterium tuberculosis
  Mycobacterium avium complex
  Pneumococcal pneumonia
  H Flu pneumonia
  Staphylococcal infection
  Recurrent pneumonia

EPIDEMIOLOGY OF HIV

- High risk factors for HIV
  homosexual/bisexual men
  IV drug abuse with needle sharing
  homosexuals who use injectable drugs
  hemophiliacs/transfusion recipients
  heterosexuals with multiple sex partners who engage in
      high risk behavior
  children born to any of the above

The CDC estimates that in the U.S. between 1 million and 1.5 million persons are infected with HIV, most of whom are asymptomatic.

HIV INFECTION IN HEALTH CARE WORKERS

Virtually all infected patients will come in contact with the health care system at some time. In the U.S. there are a small number of documented cases of occupational transmission of HIV/AIDS to health care workers. Almost all of the cases of transmission have occurred through needle sticks. A few have occurred via contact by blood with broken, unprotected skin.

SYMPTOMS OF HIV INFECTION

Within six to twelve weeks after infection with HIV, the individual may experience an acute viral syndrome characterized by: fever, lymphadenopathy, myalgia, arthralgia, diarrhea, fatigue and rash.

Sometimes infections with HIV will result in persistent, generalized lymphadenopathy (PG), a persistent swelling of the lymph nodes.

THE WINDOW PERIOD

The window period is the period of time between initial infection with HIV and seroconversion (the point at which a recently infected person begins to produce antibodies against the invading virus).

The time period may vary anywhere from two weeks to as long as three years in rare cases, but most people develop antibodies within eight to twelve weeks.

Because it is possible for a person to test negative during this window period, it is extremely important that individuals be advised not to donate blood or participate in other high risk activities, like unprotected sex, until a negative HIV status has been confirmed.

2. **Infectious Agent:** Human Immunodeficiency Virus (HIV)

3. **Incidence:** Worldwide

4. **Incubation & Period of Communicability:** The median time for onset of symptoms is eight years with an observed range of from two months to ten years from infection to the diagnosis of AIDS. The period of communicability is unknown but is presumed to begin shortly after infection and extend throughout life.

5. **Mode of Transmission:** Documented routes of transmission of HIV includes sexual intercourse; using contaminated IV needles and equipment; having parenteral, mucous membrane or non-intact skin contact with infected blood, blood components or blood products; receiving transplants of infected organs or tissues or transfusions of infected blood; through semen used for artificial insemination; and perinatal transmission (from mother to child around the time of birth). HIV virus is NOT transmitted by casual contact or by vectorborne (mosquito, tick) means.

6. **Preventive Measures:** There is no vaccine and no cure for AIDS at this time. Prevention depends on avoidance of those activities that put one at risk for acquiring infection and include: sex with someone who is infected or engages in high risk behavior; anal sex; sharing of IV needles or equipment; percutaneous, mucous membrane or non-intact skin exposure to blood and/or body fluids. Occupational exposures can be minimized by strict adherence to UNIVERSAL PRECAUTIONS, with observance of good hand washing procedure, needle and sharp precautions and appropriate use of PPE.

EXPOSURE: Extraordinary care must be taken to avoid accidental wounds from sharp instruments contaminated with potentially infective material and to avoid contact of mucous membranes and open skin lesions with material from patients. In the event of accidental percutaneous or mucosal exposure to potentially infective material from patients with HIV infection, counseling and testing should be provided to the employee. Some physicians have advocated the use of AZT very early after an exposure to a known positive source. An exposed employee should be counseled about the theoretical rationale for post exposure prophylaxis, risks of HIV infection, efficacy and toxicity of the drug and the need for follow up regardless of whether AZT is given or not.

ILLNESS: If an employee is diagnosed as having HIV/AIDS, the agency will evaluate the employee with HIV/AIDS on an ongoing basis. It is encouraged that each agency set up an expert panel. Each employee will be reviewed on a case by case basis. The expert panel will decide at what point the individual is no longer able to continue working because of work habits and severity of illness.

Isolation Code: Blood & Body Fluid Precautions

Preventive: None

B. HEPATITIS B

1. **Identification:** Disease in which the virus infects and replicates in the liver. Infection can result in one of two types of outcome–self-limited, acute hepatitis B or chronic HBV infection.

    Self-limited, acute Hepatitis B: Hepatitis B virus enters the body and attacks and infects the liver. Infection with the virus can be identified by testing for the presence of hepatitis B surface antigen (HBsAg) and/or hepatitis B core antigen (HBcAg) and/or hepatitis B e antigen (HBeAg). As the body responds to the presence of the hepatitis antigens, antibodies are formed. The presence of hepatitis B surface antibodies (Anti-HBs), coincides with the destruction of infected liver cells, elimination of the virus from the body and signifies lifetime immunity to the virus. It is this destruction of liver cells that is responsible for most of the symptoms observed. The onset of symptoms is often insidious. Severity of symptoms ranges from no symptoms to a very mild flu-like to the most severe that includes jaundice, dark urine, extreme fatigue, anorexia, nausea, abdominal pain, joint pain, rash and fever. These more severe symptoms can result in hospitalization and extended recuperation times. One to two percent of all acute hepatitis B cases will develop fulminant hepatitis which is about 85% fatal. Chronic HBV infection has more severe long term consequences. In this situation the individual does not develop antibodies to the HBsAg and cannot clear the virus from his liver. As a ~result he becomes a lifelong carrier of the virus. Such persons are at high risk for developing chronic, persistent hepatitis, cirrhosis of the liver and primary liver cancer. Pregnant women who are chronic carriers and test positive for HBeAg at time of delivery are very likely to pass on infection to their newborn.

Employee Exposure & Illness

2. **Infectious Agent:** Hepatitis B Virus (HBV)

3. **Incidence:** Worldwide

4. **Incubation & Period of Communicability:** Incubation is usually between 45-180 days, but may be as short as two weeks or as long as 6-9 months. This variation is related to the amount of virus present in the fluid, mode of transmission and host factors. Individuals can be infectious for many weeks prior to onset of symptoms, throughout the acute clinical course and during chronic carrier states. An individual is no longer considered infectious when testing indicates the presence of anti-HBs and absence of antigen (HBeAg).

5. **Mode of Transmission:** Exposure to blood and/or body fluids via percutaneous needlesticks, perinatal exposure, sexual intercourse, transfusions of unscreened or untreated blood or blood components, contact with non-intact skin or mucous membrane. Household contacts have developed infection after sharing common items such as razors or toothbrushes.

6. **Preventive Measures:** Two types of vaccine are available. Both have been shown to be safe and highly effective. One is a plasma-derived vaccine prepared from the plasma of chronic carriers. The second type of vaccine is made by recombinant DNA technology. Both types of vaccines are given in 3 IM doses, initially and 1 and 6 months later. CDC recommends the vaccine be given to those individuals at high risk of infection including occupational exposure. OSHA requires employers to provide hepatitis B vaccine at no charge to all employees at risk for occupational exposure. Recommendations for post-exposure prophylaxis is fully described in the CDC publication, MMWR February 9, 1990, Vol 39, No. RR-22. HBV carriers should be cautioned regarding their need to avoid conditions that put them at risk to transmit the virus to other individuals.

EXPOSURE: SEE ALGORITHM FOR EMPLOYEES EXPOSED TO BLOOD OR BODY FLUIDS AT THE END OF THIS SECTION.

ILLNESS: Employees diagnosed to have Hepatitis B will be off work until their symptoms subside and their HBsAg (blood test) becomes negative. If the HBsAg remains positive for over 6 months, further counseling will be needed from the expert panel. Although cautious medical personnel who are HBsAg positive have not been shown to transmit the disease, the potential liability of their employment makes many attorneys advise against it.

Isolation Code: Blood & body fluids precautions.

Preventive: Hepatitis B vaccine.

DELTA HEPATITIS

1. **Identification:** Onset is usually abrupt. Signs and symptoms are similar to Hepatitis B and is always coexistent with Hepatitis B infection. Diagnosis is made by testing for antigen and/or antibody.

2. **Infectious Agent:** Delta Hepatitis Virus

3. **Incidence:** Worldwide

4. **Incubation & Period of Communicability:** Unknown in man; blood is potentially infectious through all phases of infection.

5. **Mode of Transmission:** Same as for Hepatitis B.

6. **Preventive Measures:** No vaccine and no treatment at this time. Universal Precautions as for Hepatitis B.

EXPOSURE: See Hepatitis B

ILLNESS: See Hepatitis B

Isolation Code: Blood & Body Fluid Precautions

Preventive: None but immunity to Hepatitis B eliminates risk of Delta.

HEPATITIS C

1. **Identification:** Same as for Hepatitis B, with recent development of a test for antibody to hepatitis C, but diagnosis is usually dependent upon elimination of all other causes of disease.

2. **Infectious Agent:** Hepatitis C Virus (HCV)

3. **Incidence:** Worldwide

4. **Incubation & Period of Communicability:** Incubation is usually 2 weeks to 6 months. It is communicable from one or more weeks prior to appearance of symptoms, throughout the acute clinical course, and indefinitely in carrier states.

5. **Mode of Transmission:** Primarily through transfusions of blood but can be transmitted to health care workers through blood exposures the same as for Hepatitis B.

6. **Preventive Measures:** Same as non-A, non-B hepatitis, no vaccine available.

EXPOSURE: See Algorithm.

ILLNESS: Employees diagnosed with Hepatitis C will remain off work until symptoms subside and physician clears them to return to work

Isolation Code: Blood & Body Fluid Precautions

Preventive: None

NON-A, NON-B HEPATITIS

1. **Identification:** Causative agent not yet identified; therefore, no vaccine available. Most similar to Hepatitis B in manifestations and transmission.

2. **Infectious Agent:** Unknown but probably more than one; diagnosis is made in absence of hepatitis A or hepatitis B virus. Hepatitis C and hepatitis E virus are included.

3. **Incidence:** Worldwide

4. **Incubation & Period of Communicability:** Probably similar Hepatitis B.

5. **Mode of Transmission:** Same as for Hepatitis B.

6. **Preventive Measures:** No vaccine is available. Universal Precautions for Hepatitis B are recommended. For persons exposed to known non-A, non-B infected blood, CDC considers it reasonable to give immune globulin (IG) as treatment.

EXPOSURE: SEE ALGORITHM FOR EMPLOYEES EXPOSED TO BLOOD OR BODY FLUIDS AT THE END OF THIS SECTION.

ILLNESS: If employee is symptomatic, he/she will be off work during this period of time as determined by the expert panel. If asymptomatic may return to work once counseled by the expert panel and a return to work slip is signed by the physician.

Isolation Code: Blood & Body Fluid Precautions

Preventive: None

C. BABESIOSIS

1. **Identification:** A relatively rare but serious and sometimes fatal disease caused by infection with a protozoan parasite. Symptoms include fever, fatigue and anemia lasting days to months. In some cases no

symptoms are observed. Infection is confirmed by testing for presence of the parasite and by antibody testing.

2. **Infectious Agent:** Babesia microti.

3. **Incidence:** Found in USA in areas where host tick may be found. Endemic on Nantucket and other islands in Massachusetts, and Shelter Island and along Long Island Sound. Cases have been reported in Wisconsin and Connecticut. Cases due to another parasite have been reported in California and Georgia.

4. **Incubation & Period of Communicability:** Incubation period is from 1 week to 12 months. Not communicable between humans except through blood transfusions.

5. **Mode of Transmission:** Transmitted during the summer from the bite of a nympho tick found on voles and deer mice. The adult tick can be found primarily on deer but has been identified on other mammalian and avian hosts. Transmission has also occurred from blood transfusion with infected blood.

6. **Preventive Measures:** Universal Precautions.

EXPOSURE: No treatment indicated.

ILLNESS: Combined treatment with clindamycin and guinine has been effective.

Isolation Code: Blood & Body Fluid Precautions.

Preventive: None

D. BRUCELLOSIS

1. **Identification:** Bacterial illness characterized by fever, chills, sweating, arthralgia, weakness and general achiness. Confirmed by laboratory isolation of infectious organism from blood or other body tissues.

2. **Infectious Agent:** Brucella abortus, B. melitensis, B. suis, and B. canis.

3. **Incidence:** Worldwide. Primarily a disease of persons who work with infected animals or their tissues, especially veterinarians, farm workers and abattoir workers. Occasional outbreaks occur among those who consume unpasteurized milk or milk products from infected cows, sheep or goats. Annual cases in USA < 100.

4. **Incubation & Period of Communicability:** Variable from 5-60 days and longer. Communicability would have to be assumed to be pre-

Employee Exposure & Illness

sent as long as organism is in blood. Transmission from person to person is not documented except for one transfusion.

5. **Mode of Transmission:** Contact with tissues, blood, urine, vaginal discharges, aborted fetuses and especially placentas and by ingestion of raw milk or milk products from infected animals. Airborne transmission has occurred in man in laboratories and abattoirs. Transmission by blood transfusion has been documented.

6. **Preventive Measures:** Universal Precautions. Avoid consuming milk or dairy products that are untreated and/or unpasteurized.

EXPOSURE: No treatment indicated.

ILLNESS: Six week treatment of rifampin 600-900mg and doxycycline, 200mg daily, is recommended. Off work until all draining lesions have cleared.

Isolation Code: Blood & Body Fluid Precautions.

Preventive: None

E. COLORADO TICK FEVER (ARBOVIRAL INFECTION)

1. **Identification:** An acute febrile illness, characterized by diphasic fever, chills, headache, muscle and back aches, neutropenia, and thrombocytopenia. Moderately severe disease can occasionally lead to encephalitis, myocarditis or bleeding. Laboratory confirmation of virus in blood.

2. **Infectious Agent:** Viruses of Colorado Tick Fever.

3. **Incidence:** Areas above 5000 feet in western Canada, Washington, Oregon, Idaho, Montana, California, Nevada, Utah, Wyoming, Colorado, New Mexico and South Dakota. Several hundred cases are reported annually in the USA.

4. **Incubation & Period of Communicability:** Incubation is usually 4-5 days. Ticks remain infective for life. Virus can be isolated in blood from 2-16 weeks or more after onset of symptoms.

5. **Mode of Transmission:** From the bite of an infective tick. Ticks are found on small mammals. Transmission by blood transfusion has been documented.

6. **Preventive Measures:** Universal Precautions for blood and/or body fluids and avoid ticks or remove from infected patient. Avoid close contact with small animals in endemic regions.

EXPOSURE: No treatment indicated.

ILNESS: Off-work during acute illness. Excercise special precautions to prevent accidental exposure of patients or co-workers to employees blood or body fluids for at least four months.

Isolation Code: Blood & Body Fluid Precautions.

Preventive: None

F. CREUTZFELDT–JAKOB DISEASE

1. **Identification:** A very rare disease characterized by symptoms of confusion, progressive dementia, variable ataxia, myoclonic jerks, spasticity, wasting and coma. Disease progresses rapidly once symptoms begin with death occurring within 3-12 months. Diagnosis is complicated and requires exclusion of other neurological diseases or causes.

2. **Infection Agent:** Virus.

3. **Incidence:** Reported from 50 countries, rare.

4. **Incubation & Period of Communicability:** Incubation is long, from 15 months to more than 20 years in iatrogenic cases. Unknown in most cases. CNS tissues are infectious throughout illness. Other tissues and CSF may be infectious. Infectivity not known. Probably begins before symptoms begin.

5. **Mode of Transmission:** In most cases mode is unknown. Transmission has been documented from infected corneal transplant, insertion of cortical electrodes that had been used on known C-J patients, infected grafts of human dura mater, and several from injections of growth hormone prepared from human pituitary glands. Others have had history of brain or eye surgery within 2 years, and there is one case of a health care worker who became infected while working in a laboratory where she prepared brain specimens. Actual means of transmission is not known.

6. **Preventive Measures:** Universal Precautions. Careful and thorough disinfecting of instruments used on these patients.
EXPOSURE: No treatment indicated.

ILLNESS: Individuals with Creutzfeldt-Jakob infection after a prolonged incubation period will become very ill, requiring hospitalization.

Isolation Code: Blood & Body Fluid Precautions.

Preventive: None

G. VIRAL HEMORRHAGIC FEVER (LASSA, MARBURG, EBOLA, CRIMEAN-CONGO)

1. **Identification:** Severe viral illness characterized by fever, sore throat, cough, chest pain, vomiting that can progress to hemorrhage, shock, encephalopathy and death. Diagnosis is made by isolation of virus in blood, urine or throat washings.

2. **Infectious Agent:** Lassa virus, Marburg virus, Ebola virus and Crimean-Congo hemorrhagic fever virus.

3. **Incidence:** None of these diseases are indigenous to the USA but may occur in persons who have traveled abroad. Lassa fever in west Africa; Marburg has been recognized in Germany, former Yugoslavia, former Uganda and Kenya; Ebola disease in the Sudan, Zaire and other areas in sub-Saharan Africa; Crimean-Congo in western Crimean and other areas of the former USSR, former Yugoslavia, Bulgaria, Iraq, the Arabian Peninsula, Pakistan, western China, tropical Africa and South Africa.

4. **Incubation & Period of Communicability:** Lassa fever incubation is usually 6-21 days. Persons are communicable while virus can be isolated in their throat, and virus has been isolated in urine up to 9 weeks after onset of illness. Marburg virus incubation is 3-9 days, and Ebola virus incubation is 2-21 days. Communicable as long as virus can be found in blood and secretions. Ebola virus has been demonstrated in semen up to the 61st day after onset of illness. Crimean-Congo virus incubation is 3-12 days. Tick probably remains infective for life.

5. **Mode of Transmission:** Lassa fever by direct or indirect contact with rodent excreta, direct contact with blood, pharyngeal secretions, urine of infected patients, and by sexual contact. Marburg disease by direct contact with infected blood, secretions, organs or semen. Nosocomial infections have been frequent. Ebola virus transmission has also occurred as a result of parenteral contact with contaminated needles and syringes with these cases always being fatal. Transmission through semen has occurred 7 weeks after clinical recovery. Crimean-congo virus is transmitted by bites from infected ticks, to medical workers after exposure to infected blood or secretions, and has occurred in association with butchering infected animals.

6. **Preventive Measures:** Stay home.* No vaccines available. Strict adherence to Universal Precautions with all patients' blood and body fluids, secretions and excretions. Careful cleaning and decontamination of all items prior to disposal or returned for reuse.

EXPOSURE: No treatment indicated. Surveillance of contacts is recommended.

ILLNESS: Appropriate anti-viral agents are recommended.

Isolation Code: Blood & Body Fluid Precautions.

Preventive: None

H. HUMAN T-LYMPHOTROPIC VIRUS TYPE I

1. **Identification:** Associated with malignant neoplasm of lymphatic tissue, leukemias and lymphomas of T-cells and with a degenerative neurologic disease known as tropical spastic paraparesis or HTLV-1 related myelopathy.

2. **Infections Agent:** HTLV-1.

3. **Incidence:** Endemic in southern Japan, Caribbean, and in some parts of Africa, but also found in USA primarily in IV drug users.

4. **Incubation & Period of Communicability:** Unknown.

5. **Mode of Transmission:** Mother to child through blood or breast milk, transfusions of blood or blood products, sharing of IV needles or equipment, and sexual transmission.

6. **Preventive Measures:** Universal Precautions. No vaccine.

EXPOSURE: No treatment indicated.

ILLNESS: No specific treatment.

Isolation Code: Blood & Body Fluid Precautions.

Preventive: None

I. LEPTOSPIROSIS

1. **Identification:** Bacterial infection with fever and sudden onset of headache, chills and severe myalgia. Other symptoms include diphasic fever, meningitis, rash, anemia, hemorrhage into skin and mucous membranes, jaundice, mental confusion/depression and pulmonary symptoms. Some cases are asymptomatic, and others are often misdiagnosed. Laboratory confirmation of presence of leptospires from blood.

2. **Infectious Agent:** Leptospira interrogans, a spirochete.

Employee Exposure & Illness

3. **Incidence:** Worldwide, especially to persons exposed to rivers, lakes or other water where infected animals urinate.

4. **Incubation & Period of Communicability:** Incubation period is usually 10 days, ranging from 4-19 days. Leptospires are excreted in urine for one month but have been demonstrated to be present for up to 11 months after acute illness.

5. **Mode of Transmission:** Skin contact (especially non-intact skin or mucous membrane with water, moist soil or vegetation contaminated with urine of infected animals or direct contact with urine or tissues of infected animals. No reported cases of transmission from nosocomial exposure to blood have occurred.

6. **Preventive Measures:** Universal Precautions. Protective outerwear when exposure to potentially infected water or soil may occur.

EXPOSURE: No treatment recommended.

ILLNESS: Appropriate antibiotic therapy. Off-work until acute illness resolves.

Isolation Code: Blood & Body Fluid Precautions.

Preventive: None

J. MALARIA

1. **Identification:** Potentially fatal illness characterized by paroxysms of fever, chills, anemia, sweats and may progress to more severe CNS symptoms including coma and other organ failures. Laboratory evidence confirms the presence of malaria parasites in the blood. The disease may manifest in intervals of symptoms occurring every day, every other day or every third day. Duration of illness in untreated persons lasts from a week to a month or longer. The disease is characterized by relapses between periods of no parasitemia. This may continue irregularly for 2 to 5 years and in some cases for up to 50 years.

2. **Infectious Agent:** Plasmodium vivax, P. malariae, P. falciparum and P. ovale.

3. **Incidence:** No longer a major problem in temperate or affluent tropical environments but does remain a problem in tropical environments where there is low socioeconomic conditions. In the late 1980s there were several outbreaks of mosquito-borne malaria in southern California.

4. **Incubation & Period of Communicability:** The time between the infective bite and the appearance of symptoms is variable depending on the organism, ranging between 12 days and 10 months or longer.

Communicability occurs as long as the organism remains in the blood. The mosquito is infectious for life.

5. **Mode of Transmission:** Mosquito-borne transmission is the primary mode. May also be transmitted through needle-sticks or transfusions or by sharing of IV needles or equipment.

6. **Preventive Measures:** Universal Precautions and prophylactic antimalarial chemotherapy when in endemic areas or exposure.

EXPOSURE: Anti-Malarial drug therapy is available.

ILLNESS: Anti-Malarial drug therapy and off-work during febrile episodes.

Isolation Code: Blood & Body Fluid Precautions.

Preventive: None at this time.

K. SYPHILIS

1. **Identification:** Following infection and an incubation period, the disease will manifest itself in three stages if untreated. The primary phase is characterized by the appearance of a single lesion (chancre), a painless lesion with serous exudate. Untreated this lesion will resolve within weeks. The secondary phase begins 4-6 weeks later with the appearance of a symmetrical maculopapular rash on the palms and soles, accompanied by fever and adenopathy. The secondary phase resolves within weeks to 12 months. The majority of patients will then go into a latency period of weeks to years. The third phase or tertiary syphilis is characterized by involvement of many body systems including skin, bones, CNS and cardiovascular system with high morbidity and mortality. Laboratory evidence of the presence of spirochetes may be demonstrated during the initial phase and throughout clinical infection, although it is markedly reduced during tertiary syphilis.

2. **Infectious Agent:** Treponema pallidum.

3. **Incidence:** Worldwide.

4. **Incubation & Period of Communicability:** Incubation period is between 10 days and 3 months. Communicability is variable and indefinite. Effective antibiotic treatment usually ends infectivity within 24-48 hours.

5. **Mode of Transmission:** Primarily sexually transmitted or in utero. However, there are documented cases of transmission by needle-stick, by tattooing instruments and by blood transfusions, or on the hands of health care workers after examining infected lesions.

6. **Preventive Measures:** No vaccine available. Same precautions as for Hepatitis B. Preventive treatment with an effective antibiotic during the incubation period would be expected to prevent manifestation of symptoms and serological test positivity.

EXPOSURE: Confirmed exposures should receive prophylactic antibiotic treatment.

ILLNESS: Off-work until all draining lesions or mucous membranes have cleared.

Isolation Code: Blood & Body Fluid Precautions.

Preventive: None.

L. RELAPSING FEVER

1. **Identification:** Rare, systemic spirochetal infection characterized by recurring fevers separated by periods of relative well-being. Transitory petechial rashes are common during initial fever. Fatality rate is 2-10% but may go as high as 50% in epidemic louse-borne infections.

2. **Infectious Agent:** Louse-borne disease = Borrelia recurrentis. In tick-borne diseases many different strains of spirochetes have been distinguished.

3. **Incidence:** Epidemic louse-borne infection has not been reported in the USA in many years. Tick-borne fever has occasionally occurred in limited areas of western states.

4. **Incubation & Period of Communicability:** Incubation is from 5-15 days. Louse becomes infective within 4-5 days after ingestion of blood from an infected person and remains so for life. Infected ticks can remain infected for life and can pass on the infection to their progeny.

5. **Mode of Transmission:** Vector-borne, transmission usually occurs while crushing an infective tick thus contaminating the bite wound or abraded skin. Transmission has also occurred when blood from an infected patient contacted mucous membrane of the nose and eyes of health care workers.

6. **Preventive Measures:** Universal Precautions. Control of lice and ticks.

EXPOSURE: Antibiotic therapy is recommended after confirmed exposure if risk of infection is high.

ILLNESS: Antibiotic (tetracycline) treatment.

Isolation Code: Blood & Body Fluid Precautions.

Preventive: None

CAMPYLOBACTER

See Gastrointestinal Illnesses, acute

CHILDHOOD DISEASES

A. CHICKENPOX (VARICELLA ZOSTER)

One of the most highly communicable diseases known to man, characterized by itchy, fluid filled lesions. May be accompanied by fever, headache and general malaise. Lesions can appear on scalp, mucous membranes and conjunctiva, but generally are more frequently found on covered parts of the body. More severe in adults than children.

Transmission occurs by direct contact, inhalation of infected droplets, and sometimes by contact with freshly contaminated articles.

Lifelong immunity occurs after initial infection, however, it is not uncommon for the virus to remain dormant in the body for years and then to resurface during periods of stress or immune system suppression. When this occurs the condition is referred to as shingles. Patients with shingles have lesions that may be localized to a specific nerve pathway such as on the chest, or the face, or lesions may be disseminated. Varicella Virus is communicable from patients with first time acute infections (chicken pox) and from shingles.

Prevention of transmission requires strict isolation of infected individuals. An infected person can transmit virus during the incubation period and throughout clinical disease until all lesions are dry.

EXPOSURE: Susceptible employees with confirmed exposure to chickenpox, draining or fluid filled zoster lesions, should be off work from the 10th through the 21st day after exposure and if infection occurs, until all lesions are dry and crusted.

Employees are considered susceptible unless they can state that they have had chicken pox. If the employee has a negative history for chickenpox, he/she should be referred for a V-Z titer. Employees with positive history or positive V-Z titer, no further action is required. Employees with negative history for chickenpox and negative V-Z titer are considered susceptible.

ILLNESS: Employees infected with chickenpox or shingles (Varicella Zoster) should remain off work until all lesions are dry and crusted.

NOTE: Period of communicability for chickenpox begins two days before onset of rash and lasts until at least seven days after the first crop of vesicles have appeared and all lesions have crusted. Varicella Zoster is communicable while lesions are fluid filled, draining lesions or vesicles are present. Exposure can be by airborne, direct contact or indirect contact, thus these patients are maintained to strict isolation.

Isolation Code: Strict

Preventive: None

B. MEASLES (RUBEOLA, HARD MEASLES, 7-DAY MEASLES, RED MEASLES)

Highly contagious viral disease characterized by early URI symptoms and Koplik spots, followed by a red, blotchy rash appearing 3-7 days later. Common complications include pneumonia, otitis media and encephalitis.

Transmission occurs by droplets or direct contact with secretions from mouth or nose. Indirect transmission can occur from articles freshly contaminated by mouth and nose secretions. Airborne transmission can occur.

EXPOSURE: All susceptible employees exposed to known measles cases should be off work from the 5th through the 21st day after exposure and/or until 7 days after the rash appears.

Susceptible personnel: All persons born prior to 1957 have probably been infected naturally and generally need not be considered susceptible. Employees born after 1957 can be considered immune only if documentation of:
1. physician-diagnosed measles;
2. laboratory evidence of measles immunity (titer);
3. adequate immunization with two doses of live measles vaccine 30 days apart after their first birthday.

ILLNESS: Employees diagnosed with measles will remain off work until 7 days after the rash appears.

Isolation Code: Respiratory Isolation and Contact Isolation.

Preventive: 2 doses of live measles vaccine 30 days apart after first birthday. MMR vaccine is recommended, as it offers protection for both forms of measles, as well as mumps.

C. MUMPS

Acute viral infection characterized by painful swelling of parotid gland and usually accompanied by fever. Complications include infection of the testes, ovaries, aseptic meningitis, rarely deafness. Infection of other organs or body systems can occur including joints, nerves, pancreas, heart, thyroid gland, and kidneys.

Transmission occurs via droplet spread or by direct contact with infected saliva.

EXPOSURE: All employees with a positive history of mumps or those with a history of having received mumps vaccination can be considered immune.

Susceptible employees should remain off work from the 12th through the 26th day after exposure or until 9 days after onset of parotitis.

ILLNESS: Personnel who develop symptoms of mumps will be off work until 9 days after the onset of parotitis (swollen parotid gland).

Isolation Code: Respiratory and Contact Isolation.

Preventive: Live mumps vaccine is recommended. MMR is the vaccine of choice if employee is likely to be susceptible to measles and rubella.

D. RUBELLA (GERMAN MEASLES – THREE DAY MEASLES)

Highly contagious viral infection which produces a mild febrile disease characterized by a pink pinpoint rash. Greatest hazard is to a fetus during the first trimester when congenital defects, abortion and stillbirth can result. Other complications from Rubella infection include arthritis and rarely encephalitis.

Transmission occurs via droplet spread, direct contact with infected person or by indirect contact with articles contaminated with oral or nasal secretions, blood, urine or feces. Strict isolation is recommended with good handwashing technique, and when close contact may occur, a mask and eyewear may be worn to prevent droplet spread to the mucous membranes of the nose, mouth and eyes.

EXPOSURE: Susceptible employees exposed to patients with confirmed rubella during the communicable period and when respiratory isolation precautions have not been followed or in the case of congenital, when strict isolation has not been followed will be removed from work from the 7th to the 21st day after exposure and/or 5 days after the rash appears.

Employees are to be considered susceptible unless they have documentation of:

1. laboratory evidence of immunity (rubella titer greater than 1 to 8, values may vary with lab);

2. immunization with live virus vaccine on or after first birthday.

ILLNESS: Employees with diagnosed rubella will remain off work until 5 days after rash appears.

Isolation Code: Contact/Respiratory/Strict

Preventive: Single dose of live, attenuated rubella vaccine. MMR is vaccine of choice if employee is likely to be susceptible to measles and/or mumps.

E. PERTUSSIS (WHOOPING COUGH)

Bacterial infection most common in young children. Characterized by classic paroxysmal coughing followed by rapid, deep inspiration accompanied by whooping or crowing sound. Mucus induced gagging and choking often occurs. Paroxysmal stage lasts three weeks to two months. These children look and sound as ill as they are, but fatality is low. Contagious as long as three weeks after onset if no treatment is given.

Transmission occurs via airborne route or direct contact with oral or nasal secretions.

EXPOSURE: Antimicrobial prophylaxis against pertussis should be offered immediately to susceptible personnel who have had intensive contact with an infected patient without using proper precautions.

Pertussis vaccine is not recommended for adults.

ILLNESS: Those employees with active pertussis should not be allowed to work from the beginning of the catarrhal stage through the third week after onset of paroxysms or until seven (7) days after the start of effective therapy.

During an outbreak, personnel with cough or upper respiratory tract symptoms should not perform patient care.

Isolation Code: Respiratory Isolation

Preventive: Adults - none recommended; Children - Pertussis vaccine.

COMMON COLD/VIRAL UPPER RESPIRATORY INFECTION

Characterized by cough, sneezing, itching watery eyes, raspy throat, headache, general malaise, and low grade fever. Symptoms usually develop within 12-72 hours after exposure and last 2-7 days.

Causative agent is any of a number of viruses including rhino viruses (over 100) and influenza viruses as well as others.

Transmission can occur in several ways depending on the particular virus. Respiratory transmission occurs when droplet nuclei are inhaled or by direct contact when larger droplets are sprayed directly into the mouth, nose and eyes during talking, coughing or sneezing. Indirect contact can occur when the hands become contaminated by infected droplets or by handling of dried secretions and then touching the mucous membranes of the eyes or mouth.

Prevention of transmission includes wearing of masks/eye protection when in close contact with patients with respiratory symptoms and rigorous handwashing policies. Hands should be washed before and after all patient contact and after handling patients' items, especially those that may be soiled with respiratory secretions. EMS personnel should always wash their hands prior to eating, smoking or touching the face.

EXPOSURE: No treatment indicated.

ILLNESS: Infected health care workers should avoid patient contact or wear a mask when in close contact with patients or other employees. Masks should be changed frequently and anytime they become moisture laden.

Isolation Code: Contact and wear mask if close contact.

Preventive: None, although flu vaccine may offer some protection during periods of outbreak.

CONJUNCTIVITIS - INFECTIOUS AND DRAINING (PINK EYE)

Highly infectious inflammation of the conjunctiva of one or both eyes. Symptoms include tearing, itching, sensitivity to light, and purulent discharge.

Transmission is by direct or indirect contact with discharge from eyes or respiratory tract of infected persons. Several causative agents both bacterial and viral. Good handwashing technique is very important in preventing transmission.

Infectious Agent: Most often staphylococous, streptococcus, hemophitus and pseudomonas bacteria.

EXPOSURE: No treatment indicated. Careful handwashing is the best means to prevent the spread of infection.

ILLNESS: Employees with active conjunctivitis and drainage should not be allowed to work until the discharge ceases.

Isolation Code: Contact - very easily spread unless strict adherence to contact isolation techniques.

Preventive: None

CMV - CYTOMEGALIC VIRUS

A viral infection which is usually asymptomatic except in the perinatal period, when consequences to the fetus may be severe. Susceptibility increases with pregnancy, debilitation, immunosuppressive drug therapy, and HIV infection.

EXPOSURE: No specific treatment indicated. Careful hand washing after exposure is the most effective means of preventing transmission of disease.

ILLNESS: Personnel who contract illness thought to be due to CMV need not be restricted from work. Careful hand washing and exercising care to prevent their body fluids from contacting other persons should be observed.

Isolation Code: Contact isolation precautions.

Preventive: None

DIPHTHERIA

Diphtheria - Acute upper respiratory infection, with expected symptoms and swelling of the throat. Grayish-white patches/pseudomembrane may be apparent on the mucous membranes of the pharynx, tonsils, nose and/or larynx. Toxogenic strains cause severe and fatal cases.
Transmission occurs through direct contact with a patient or carrier. Indirect contact with articles contaminated with discharge from lesions can occur.

EXPOSURE: Susceptible persons should be followed closely. Employees vaccinated in last 10 years, no further treatment or restrictions. If vaccinated, but no booster received in last 10 years, booster dose of Td.

ILLNESS: Employees infected with diphtheria should not be permitted to work until the disease has resolved and they are deemed non-infectious by physician. This disease is an incapacitating illness and will result in hospitalization for the treatment.

Isolation Code: Strict.

Preventive: Td vaccine every 10 years.

GASTROINTESTINAL ILLNESS (ACUTE DIARRHEA/VOMITING)

Characterized by loose, watery stools, fever, and vomiting. Can be caused by a number of organisms including viruses, bacteria and parasites. Symptoms may be mild or severe and if untreated can lead to dehydration, coma and death, especially in the very young and the elderly. Organisms of particular concern include salmonella, shigella, giardia, and campylobacter.

Transmission occurs most often by fecal contamination of food, water or articles, or direct contact person to person. Poor handwashing after patient contact, or contact with articles in patient's environment and poor personal hygiene contribute to transmission.

EXPOSURE: No treatment indicated, however, should be counseled to immediately report any gastrointestinal symptoms to their supervisor.

ILLNESS: If an individual contracts an acute diarrhea illness accompanied by fever, cramps, or bloody stools, they are likely to be excreting potentially infective organisms. The specific cause of acute diarrhea, however, cannot be determined solely on the basis of clinical symptoms.

Therefore:
1. A stool culture will be obtained when the above symptoms are exhibited.
2. The individual will remain off work during the febrile illness. He/she may return to work once he/she has clinically recovered.
3. If the employee is given antibiotics, a follow-up culture will be done at or over 48 hours after the last dose. If not, a culture will be done 48 hours after the individual has clinically recovered.
4. If an employee is cultured positive for salmonella, shigella, giardia, or campylobacter, he/she will be seen by the consulting physician for treatment and will not be permitted to work until five (5) days after medication has been started and three (3) negative stool cultures, not less than 24 hours apart, have been obtained.

Isolation Code: Enteric

Preventive: No vaccines recommended

GIARDIA LAMBLIA

see Gastrointestinal Illness, Acute.

HEPATITIS NON-BLOODBORNE
A. HEPATITIS A & E

This is a generally mild disease characterized by abrupt onset of symptoms and sometimes jaundice and liver enlargement. Symptoms tend to be less severe in children, more severe in adults. It is a viral disease transmitted by direct person-to-person contact with fecal contamination, and oral ingestion or transmission occurs more easily when poor handwashing techniques and poor hygiene is practiced. Incubation period is 2-6 weeks with contagion occurring late in the incubation period and into the acute illness, diminishing with onset of jaundice.

EXPOSURE: Routine IG prophylaxis is not recommended. Personnel should be counseled regarding need for good handwashing and hygiene practices and advised to contact supervisor if symptoms develop.

ILLNESS: Employees diagnosed with Hepatitis A should be off work during the symptomatic period as determined by the consulting physician. They may return to work when asymptomatic, as determined by consulting physician, once counseled by physician and a return to work form is submitted by the physician.

Isolation Code: Enteric

Preventive: None

HERPES SIMPLEX VIRUS (COLD SORES, DRAINING/HERPETIC WHITLOW)

Herpes simplex is a viral infection characterized by lesions that may appear either in the mouth area or in the genital area. These lesions start out with superficial clear vesicles which open, crust over and heal within a few days. It is worldwide in its occurrence. Incubation period is from 2-12 days. Reactivation is precipitated by a number of factors, some of which may be stress, some dietary foods, rays from the sun, etc. Recurrence is frequently characterized by discomfort in the area where the sore will appear, burning, itching, tingling. Generally we understand herpes to be in the mouth area or in the genital region, but in the course of health care delivery one also needs to be concerned with Herpetic Whitlow. It too is herpes but usually on the fingers of the health care person contracted through exposure from oral secretions of infected patients.

Direct contact with the virus in the saliva or through sexual contact is probably the most important mode of spread. Individuals with herpes lesions are usually capable of spreading the virus for up to 7-12 days or until all lesions are dried and crusted. Health personnel should therefore wear gloves whenever in direct contact with potentially infectious lesions.

EXPOSURE: If an employee is exposed to a patient with known or suspected herpes simplex and:

1. infection control guidelines were followed, no further action is needed;

2. infection control guidelines were not followed, an exposure report should be generated, however, no treatment is indicated.

ILLNESS: Employees with draining cold sores or herpetic lesions on the hands or fingers should not be permitted to engage in direct patient care. Lesions on other areas of the body can be contained within an appropriate barrier such as mask or gauze dressing. If drainage cannot be contained within the barrier, the employee will not be permitted to work until lesions are dry and crusted and no drainage is evident.

Isolation Code: Primary or disseminated - Strict

Recurrent - Drainage/Secretion

Preventive: None

MENINGITIS

Infection of the meninges surrounding the brain. Caused by viruses, bacteria and on occasion amoeba. Symptoms may include headache, photophobia, irritability, muscular rigidity, fever, weakness, malaise, personality changes, seizures, coma, shock, vomiting and lethargy.

Mode of transmission is dependent upon causative agent. However, because causative agent is usually unknown, preventive measures should be followed assuming respiratory and direct contact transmission.

Viral infections: Usually less severe and self-limiting infections. See causative agents such as mumps, measles, rubella, herpes for Exposure and Illness recommendations.

Bacterial infections: Rapid onset of symptoms, often severe but if treated early will usually respond to antibiotic therapy. For exposure and illness recommendations, see below.

A. MENINGOCOCCAL MENINGITIS/SEPTICEMIA

EXPOSURE: Antimicrobial prophylaxis should be offered immediately to employees who have had droplet contact with an infected patient. If treatment is deemed necessary, treatment should not await results of antimicrobial sensitivity testing. The following regimes may be considered for prophylaxis of adults in the following order of preference:

1. Rifampin, 600 mg orally twice daily for two days.

2. Minocycline, 100-200 mg orally every 12 hours for three days.

3. Sulfonamides should be administered only if the organism has been demonstrated to be sulfa sensitive.

NOTE: Individuals previously treated with Rifampin shall be referred to the consulting physician for evaluation and determination of most appropriate therapy prior to a subsequent treatment.

ILLNESS: Employees with active meningococcal disease should not be permitted to work until complete resolution of the disease.

Isolation Code: Respiratory Isolation

Preventive: None

B. HAEMOPHILUS MENINGITIS (H-Flu)

EXPOSURE: Observation recommended. In some cases prophylactive Rifampin 20 mg/kg orally once/day for four days may be considered.

ILLNESS: Ill employees should not be permitted to work until complete resolution of disease.

Isolation Code: Respiratory Isolation

Preventive: Vaccine for children, and for persons at risk for fatal infection

PLAGUE

A. BUBONIC AND PNEUMONIC

A bacterial infection that usually involves lymph nodes (Bubonic) but may progress to septicemia, with meningeal infection and lung involvement causing pneumonia, pleural effusion and mediastinal infections. Pneumonic plague is especially significant in that it has a high fatality rate and can lead to airborne transmission through aerosolized droplets.

Transmission: Infected fleas that live on wild rodents such as ground squirrels, rabbits and occasionally domestic cats or urban rats have been sources of infections in humans. Pneumonic Plague can be spread from person to person via airborne route. EMS personnel should avoid contact with wild rodents, especially ground squirrels and animals that reside where the disease is prevalent in these animals. These areas are often identified and posted by local health departments during periods of outbreaks.

Transmission can occur after treating/transporting an infected person and infected fleas remain in linens or other articles, or these items have been contaminated with pus from buboes.

EXPOSURE: EMS personnel with known exposure to vectors should be disinfected by spraying with an appropriate insecticide. All close contacts should be evaluated for chemotherapy. Personnel exposed to known or suspected pneumonic cases should be treated with tetracycline (15-30 mg/kg) or sulfanomides (40 mg/kg) daily in four divided doses for one week.

Isolation: Pneumonic - Strict; Bubonic - Contact

Preventive: None

PNEUMONIA

Infection of the lungs characterized by fever, chills, dyspnea, cough (often productive and pleural (chest) pain. Wheezes and rales may also be present. Pneumonia is a leading important cause of death in infants and elderly. Causative agents include pneumococcal, mycoplasma, pneumocystis carinii, chlamydia, TWAR agent, and numerous viruses.

Transmission occurs through droplets, direct contact with oral and nasal secretions and from indirect contact with articles contaminated with oral and nasal discharges.

EXPOSURE: No treatment recommended.

ILLNESS: Employee should remain off work until symptoms have resolved and after initiation of effective antibiotic treatment.

Isolation Code: Respiratory and contact.

Preventives: Polyvalent vaccine available for pneumococcal infections recommended for high risk persons such as those with compromised immune systems.

RABIES

Acute viral disease of the central nervous system; almost always fatal. Symptoms include fever, headache, restlessness and mental depression, progressing to paresis or paralysis, spasms of muscles involved in swallowing leading to fear of water. Respiratory depression ultimately causes death, usually within a week or so. Rare in humans.

Transmission occurs when saliva from an infected animal (human) enters a wound, a bite, scratch, or previous injury. Airborne transmission has occurred in cases where millions of infected bats reside.

EXPOSURE: EMS personnel bitten or scratched by an animal or having non-intact skin that has contacted animal or infected human's saliva should:

1. Immediately and thoroughly cleanse the wound with soap and copious flushing with water.

2. Thorough cleansing of wounds by medical personnel.

3. Rabies immune globulin (RIG) and/or vaccine as indicated. RIG is given, half of dose infiltrated at wound site and the rest IM. Vaccine is given in 5 doses, 1 immediately, other doses at 3, 7, 14 and 28-35 days. Decision to administer

RIG or vaccine will be dependent on type of animal, nature of attack (provoked vs. unprovoked), whether animal is available for examination, and incidence of rabies in area and species.

4. Tetanus prophylaxis and antibacterial treatment when required.

5. No sutures or wound closure is advised unless unavoidable, and then should be done loosely permitting free drainage from wound. Recommendations are from Control of Communicable Diseases In Man, 15th Edition 1990. A.S. Benenson, Editor.

Isolation: Strict isolation.

Preventive: Vaccine is available for high risk professions such as veterinarian, conservation officers, and park rangers in enzootic areas, etc. EMS personnel are not included in this group.

SALMONELIA

see Gastrointestinal Illness, Acute

SCABIES

Infectious skin disease caused by parasitic mites who burrow into the skin and deposit eggs. May be seen as small burrow lines, especially in skin folds. Lesions cause intense itching and when scratched, often lead to secondary infections. Transmitted skin to skin, especially venereally. Incubation period is from 2-8 weeks before onset of itching is primary exposure. Persons previously infected develop symptoms 1-10 days after re-exposure or re-infection.

EXPOSURE: Susceptible employees having no symptoms of scabies but with a history of casual skin contact with scabitic person should be permitted to continue working and will be treated prophylactically with anti-scabicide (Kwell) at the discretion of the consulting physician.

ILLNESS: Employees with minor symptoms and a history of close skin contact with scabitic person will be excluded from work until treated with anti-scabicide (Kwell) by the consulting physician.

Employees with suspected community exposure to scabies and who are infested with the mite should be excluded from work until they are treated.

Isolation Code: Contact

Preventive: No vaccine

SHIGELIA

see Gastrointestinal Illness, Acute

STAPHYLOCOCCUS AUREUS INFECTION AND CARRIAGE

Broad category of diseases with manifestations ranging from a single pustule to septicemia and death. Scalded skin syndrome, impetigo and endocarditis are examples of staph-caused infections. Common elements include pus-filled lesions and abscess formation. Complications include pneumonitis, septicemia, brain abscess and frequently appear in patients who have debilitating illnesses or who have undergone prolonged hospitalization.

Transmission occurs by contact with a lesion or with an asymptomatic carrier. Auto-infection may account for 30 percent of cases. Most likely to occur where poor personal hygiene is practiced. Incubation varies according to type but averages 4-10 days.

EXPOSURE: No treatment indicated. Good handwashing technique is most effective means of preventing transmission.

ILLNESS: Individuals with skin infection caused by this organism will not be allowed to work until the infection is resolved. If certain individuals are linked epidemiologically to an increased number of infections, these persons will be cultured and, if positive, will be removed from patient contact until carriage is eradicated.

Isolation Code: Varies according to symptoms but generally Contact, unless respiratory component and then Strict Isolation precautions should be observed.

Preventive: None

SPECIAL NOTE: MRSA (Multidrug Resistant Staph Aureus) is a particularly difficult form of staph to eradicate. Its name implies that many of the drugs used to treat staph infections are ineffective with these strains.

EXPOSURE: No treatment or restrictions indicated. When respiratory component involved, nasopharyngeal cultures of exposed personnel may be indicated to permit treatment to eradicate carriage.

ILLNESS: Employees infected with MRSA should be excluded from work until illness resolves.

STREP THROAT GROUP A BETA STREPTOCOCCAL INFECTION

Acute streptococcal pharyngitis characterized by fever, sore throat and enlarged, tender cervical nodes. Complications from infections with strep include otitis media, acute glomerulonephritis, rheumatic fever, and rheumatic heart disease. (Streptococcal infections may also involve the skin as in pyoderma and impetigo, scarlet fever, and erysipilas, an acute cellulitis.)

Transmission is by close, direct contact especially from individuals who are nasal carriers.

EXPOSURE: No specific treatment is indicated.

ILLNESS: If an employee is cultured positive, he/she should be asked to take treatment and should remain off work until 24 hours after effective therapy has been initiated. If an employee is linked epidemiologically to the occurrence of disease, she/he should be cultured and, if positive, removed from patient contact until carriage is eradicated.

Isolation Code: Contact Isolation Precautions - wear mask if close contact with patient.

Preventive: None

TETANUS (LOCKJAW)

Anaerobic bacterial infection occurs at wound site and produces a neurotoxin which is responsible for muscle rigidity and muscle contractions. Most cases occur after minor injuries in people who have not been adequately vaccinated. Fatality rate reaches 90 percent.

Transmission occurs when tetanus spores enter a wound through contaminated soil, street dust or feces (human or animal). Incubation period is usually 3-21 days but may occur in 1 day or over several months.

EXPOSURE: MMWR Summary Guide to Tetanus Prophylaxis in Routine Wound Management

History of tetanus immunization (doses)	Clean, minor wounds		All other wounds	
	Td*	TIG†	Td*	TIG†
Uncertain	Yes	No	Yes	Yes
0-1	Yes	No	Yes	Yes
2	Yes	No	Yes	No§
3 or more	No¶	No	No**	No

NOTE: Refer to text on specific vaccines or toxoids for contraindications, precautions, dosages, side effects and adverse reactions and special considerations. Important details are in the text and ACIP recommendation (MMWR 1981; 30:392-407).

* The combined preparations Td, containing both tetanus and diptheria toxoids, is preferred to tetanus toxoid alone.
† Tetanus immune globulin.
§ Yes, if wound more than 24 hours old.
¶ Yes, if more than 10 years since last dose.
** Yes, if more than 5 years since last dose (more frequent boosters are not needed and can accentuate side effects).

ILLNESS: Employees diagnosed with tetanus should not be permitted to work until the disease has resolved and they are deemed non-infectious by consulting physician. This disease is an incapacitating illness and will result in hospitalization for treatment.

Isolation Code: None

Preventive: Td Vaccine

TUBERCULOSIS (TB)

Acute or chronic infection caused by more than a dozen strains of bacteria. Symptoms include fever, dyspnea, productive cough, often with blood-tinged sputum, weight loss and chest pain. If untreated or inadequately treated, the disease may flare up repeatedly for years. Rarely fatal if properly treated. Transmission is by airborne route. Droplet nuclei from infected person remain suspended in the air and are then inhaled. Incubation period is usually 4-12 weeks. Patients are contagious as long as the bacillus is present in sputum. Patients at greatest risk are those living in crowded, unsanitary conditions and those suffering from malnutrition, general debilitation and alcoholism.

EXPOSURE: Employees exposed to confirmed active pulmonary TB and if respiratory precautions were not followed:

1. A baseline skin test should be done as soon as possible unless the individual has had one within the last ten weeks.

2. A repeat skin test should be done ten (10) weeks after the exposure.

3. Those who have a significant reaction upon testing should be referred to the local Public Health Department or to a consulting physician for follow-up and treatment.

4. Individuals refusing preventive treatment will be counseled about the risk of developing disease and the risks they may pose to their contacts. They

should be encouraged to seek evaluation should signs and symptoms that may be due to TB occur. Document if treatment is refused.

NOTE: Those already known to have significant reactions need not be tested unless they have pulmonary symptoms that may be due to tuberculosis, and then a chest X-ray will be obtained.

ILLNESS: Personnel with current pulmonary or laryngeal TB, documented by positive AFB smears, will be excluded from work until adequate treatment has begin and the sputum is free of bacilli on three consecutive smears, obtained on separate days or until sputum cultures have no growth.

Personnel who have current TB at a site other than the lung or larynx will be allowed to continue their usual activities.

Personnel who discontinue medications before the recommended course of therapy has been completed will not be allowed to work.

Personnel who have completed preventive treatment or adequate therapy for current disease will be exempt from further screening unless symptomatic.

Isolation Code: Respiratory Isolation

When tolerated, have patient wear mask. If patient does not wear a mask, health care worker should wear a respirator (PR). CDC guidelines regarding appropriate airborne protection should be followed.

Preventive: None

WOUND INFECTIONS

Any open wound with discharge should be considered infectious and universal precautions observed. Infectious agents may be viral (i.e. herpes simplex), or bacterial (i.e. tetanus, staphylococcus, clostridium/gangrene). EMS personnel should carefully cover draining wounds to contain the drainage.

EXPOSURE: No treatment indicated. Universal precautions and good handwashing are most effective means to prevent transmission.

ILLNESS: Employees with infected wounds or lesions should be restricted from patient care contact unless drainage can be contained. Employees with draining or weeping lesions or wounds on the hands should be excluded from patient contact.

Isolation Code: Drainage/Secretion and Blood & Body Fluids Precaution.

Preventive: None

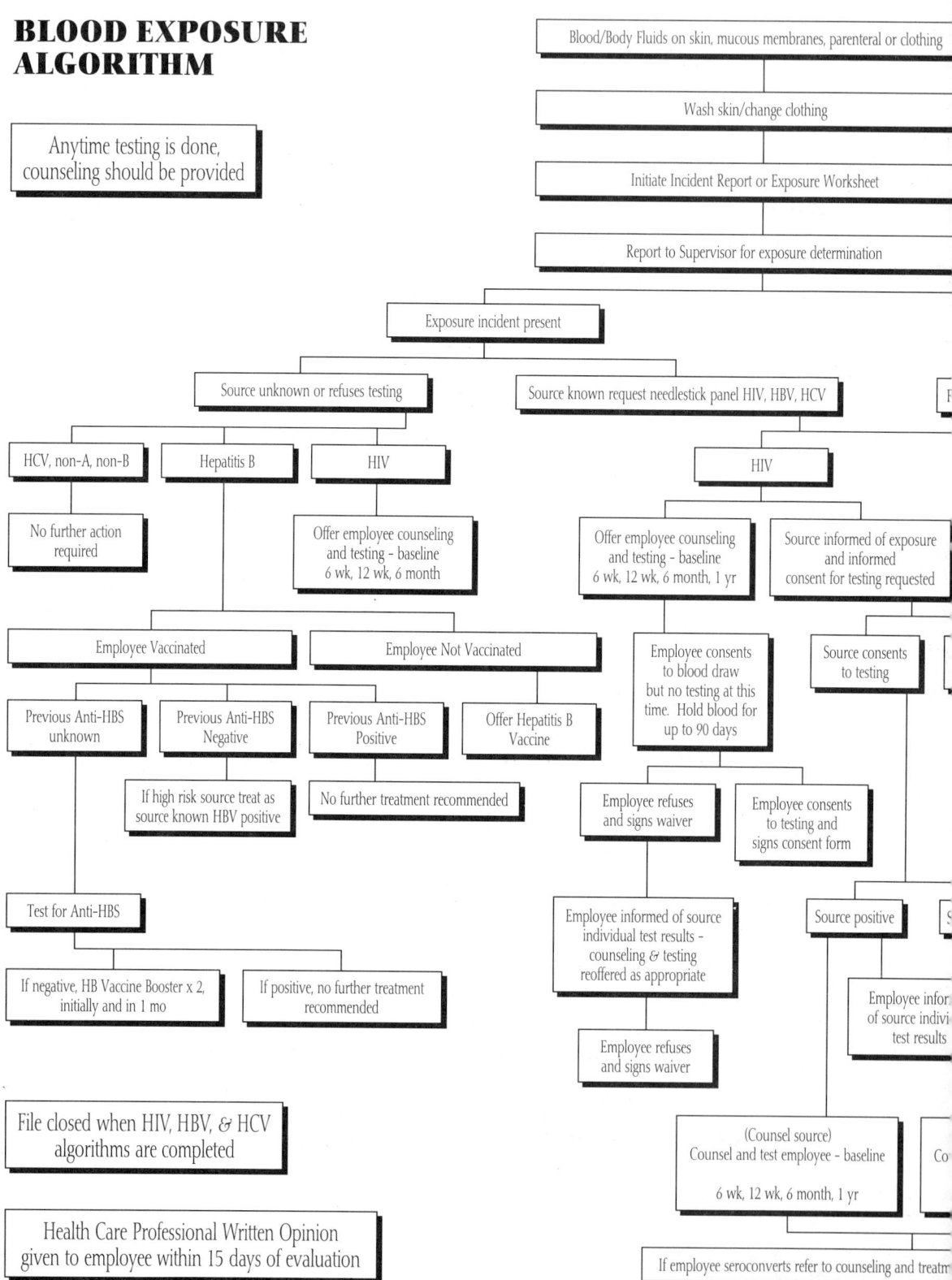

Employee Exposure & Illness 113

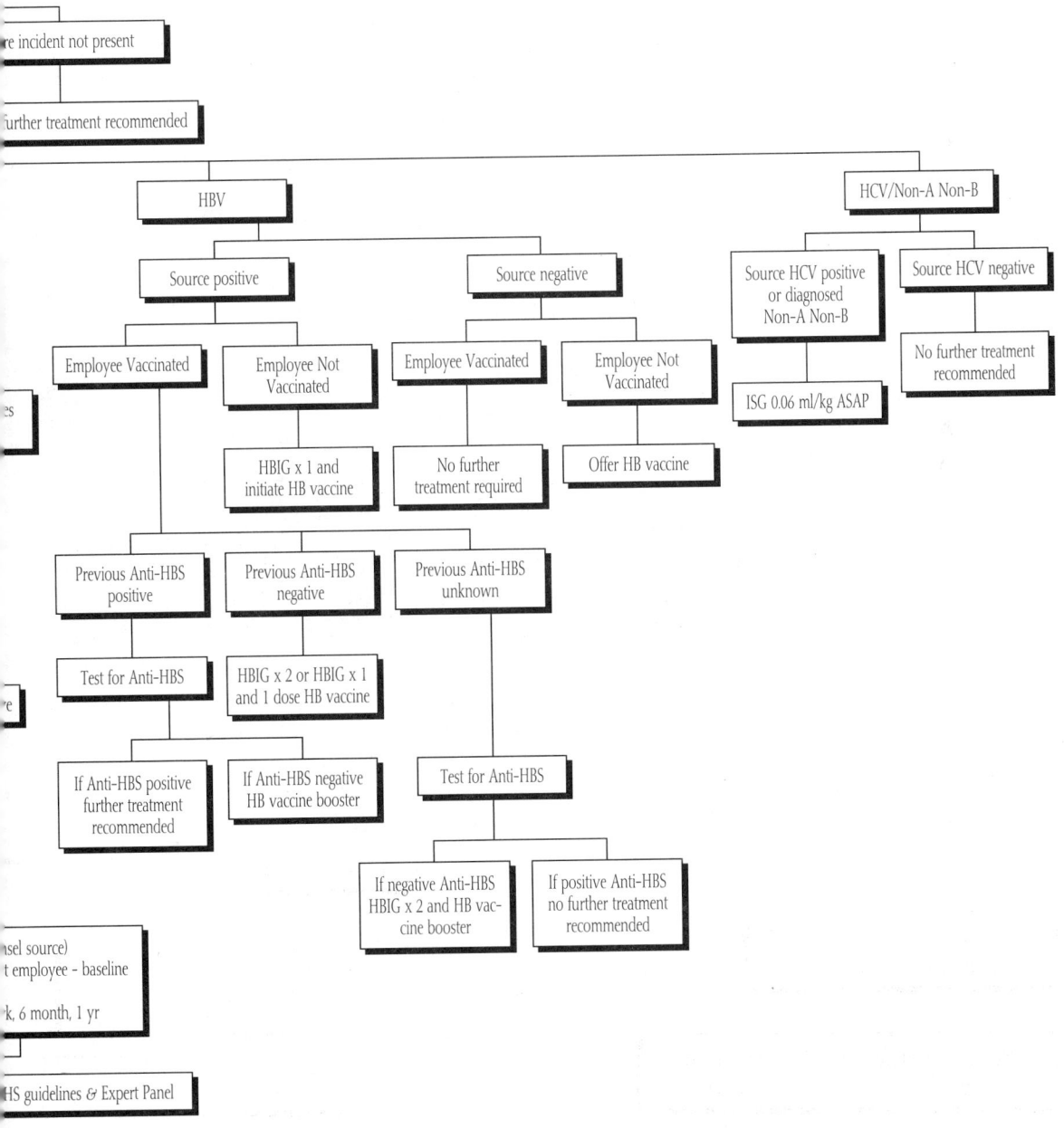

NOTES

SPECIAL SECTION

HEALTH CARE WORKERS WITH CHRONIC OR LIFE-THREATENING COMMUNICABLE DISEASES

Individuals who have entered the health care field have done so with the knowledge that there are some risks associated with this profession. Emergency medical personnel have long been exposed to the violence in our society and the stress of caring for the very ill and dying. All medical professionals know they will be caring for and therefore exposed to individuals who are ill with communicable diseases.

With the recognition of AIDS and Hepatitis B as diseases transmissible through contact with blood and certain body fluids, the concern for exposure to health care professionals has resulted in special rule making by the federal government via the Occupational Safety and Health Administration.

Along with the concern that these diseases could be transmitted as a result of occupational exposure, came the demand for mandatory testing of persons for HIV and HBV. The CDC published a report of a Florida dentist who was the Probable source of five patients becoming infected with HIV. The demand for mandatory testing became a national issue.

Follow-up reports from the CDC, indicating that a retrospective study of 15,795 patients of 2 HIV infected health care workers demonstrated no HIV infections that could be attributed to dental or medical care, received far less coverage.

While the debate continues over the value versus cost versus adverse effects that mandatory testing would cause, the CDC has published recommendations for health care settings to prevent transmission of bloodborne disease during exposure-prone, invasive procedures. Those recommendations are included here.

RECOMMENDATIONS

Investigations of HIV and HBV transmission from health care workers (HCWs) to patients indicate that, when HCWs adhere to recommended infection-control procedures, the risk of transmitting HBV from an infected HCW to a patient is small, and the risk of transmitting HIV is likely to be even smaller. However, the likelihood of exposure of the patient to an HCW's blood is greater for certain procedures designated as exposure-prone. To minimize the risk of HIV or HBV transmission, the following measures are recommended:

- All HCWs should adhere to universal precautions, including the appropriate use of hand washing, protective barriers, and care in the use and disposal of needles and other sharp instruments. HCWs who have exudative lesions or weeping dermatitis should refrain from all direct patient care and from handling patient-care equipment and devices used in performing invasive procedures until the condition resolves. HCWs should also comply with current guidelines for disinfection and sterilization of reusable devices used in invasive procedures.

- Currently available data provide no basis for recommendations to restrict the practice of HCWs infected with HIV or HBV who perform invasive procedures not identified as exposure-prone, provided the infected HCWs practice recommended surgical or dental technique and comply with universal precautions and current recommendations for sterilization/disinfection.

- Exposure prone procedures should be identified by medical/surgical/dental organizations and institutions at which the procedures are performed.

- HCWs who perform exposure-prone procedures and who do not have serologic evidence of immunity to HBV from vaccination or from previous infection should know their HBsAg status and, if that is positive, should also know their HBeAg status.

- HCWs who are infected with HIV or HBV (and are HBeAg positive) should not perform exposure-prone procedures unless they have sought counsel from an expert review panel and been advised under what circumstances, if any, they may continue to perform these procedures.* Such circumstances would include notifying prospective patients of the HCW's seropositivity before they undergo exposure-prone invasive procedures.

*The review panel should include experts who represent a balanced perspective. Such experts might include all of the following: a) the HCW's personal physician(s), b) an infectious disease specialist with expertise in the epidemiology of HIV and HBV transmission, c) a health professional with expertise in the procedures performed by the HCW, and d) state or local public health official(s). If the HCW's practice is institutionally based, the expert review panel might also include a member of the infection-control committee, preferably a hospital epidemiologist. HCWs who perform exposure-prone procedures outside the hospital/institutional setting should seek advice from appropriate state and local public health officials regarding the review process. Panels must recognize the importance of confidentiality and the privacy rights of infected HCWs.

- Mandatory testing of HCWs for HIV antibody, HBsAg, or HBeAg is not recommended. The current assessment of the risk that infected HCWs will transmit HIV or HBV to patients during exposure-prone procedures does not support the diversion of resources that would be required to implement mandatory testing programs. Compliance by HCWs with recommendations can be increased through education, training, and appropriate confidentiality safeguards.

HCWS WHOSE PRACTICES ARE MODIFIED BECAUSE OF HIV OR HBV STATUS

HCWs whose practices are modified because of their HIV or HBV infection status should, whenever possible, be provided opportunities to continue appropriate patient-care activities. Career counseling and job retraining should be encouraged to promote the continued use of the HCW's talents, knowledge, and skills. HCWs whose practices are modified because of HBV infection should be reevaluated periodically to determine whether their HBeAg status changes due to resolution of infection or as a result of treatment.

NOTIFICATION OF PATIENTS AND FOLLOW-UP STUDIES

The public health benefit of notification of patients who have had exposure-prone procedures performed by HCWs infected with HIV or positive for HBeAg should be considered on a case-by-case basis, taking into consideration an assessment of specific risks, confidentiality issues, and available resources. Carefully designed and implemented follow-up studies are necessary to determine more precisely the risk of transmission during such procedures. Decisions regarding notification and follow-up studies should be made in consultation with state and local public health officials.

ADDITIONAL NEEDS

- Clearer definition of the nature, frequency, and circumstances of blood contact between patients and HCWs during invasive procedures.

- Development and evaluation of new devices, protective barriers, and techniques that may prevent such blood contact without adversely affecting the quality of patient care.

- More information on the potential for HIV and HBV transmission through contaminated instruments.

- Improvements in sterilization and disinfection techniques for certain reusable equipment and devices.

- Identification of factors that may influence the likelihood of HIV or HBV transmission after exposure to HIV- or HBV-infected blood.

Centers for Disease Control. Recommendations for preventing transmission of human immunodeficiency virus and hepatitis B virus to patients during exposure-prone invasive procedures. MMWR 1991;40(No. RR-8): pp. 5-6

The American Ambulance Association through its Professional Standards Committee has developed a position paper regarding Health Care Professionals with chronic or life-threatening illnesses. That position paper is printed in its entirety in this chapter by permission of the American Ambulance Association, and it is hoped that organizations will adopt it for their own use.

POSITION STATEMENT OF THE AMERICAN AMBULANCE ASSOCIATION

EMPLOYEES WITH LIFE THREATENING AND/OR COMMUNICABLE ILLNESSES

The American Ambulance Association recognizes that applicants and employees with life threatening and/or communicable illnesses, including but not limited to, cancer, heart disease, AIDS (Acquired Immune Deficiency Syndrome), ARC, (AIDS Related Condition) or Hepatitis A. B. or C may wish to continue to engage in as many of their regular pursuits as their conditions allow, including work. The American Ambulance Association believes that such as employee should be permitted to do so as long as the individual is able to perform satisfactorily, and the best available medical evidence indicates that the individual's condition does not pose a direct threat to the health or safety of the individual or others. The American Ambulance Association urges all of its members to be sensitive to the conditions of such applicants and employees, and make every effort to treat them consistently with all other applicants and employees pursuant to the following guidelines:

1. Members must provide a safe work environment for employees and safe treatment for patients. Accordingly, reasonable precautions must be taken to ensure that an employee's condition does not present a health or safety risk to himself/herself, other employees, patients or others. Accordingly, members must develop and maintain effective health and safety policies, including those addressing infection and exposure control. All employees must follow the member's health and safety policies.

2. All members should be sensitive to the fact that continued employment for individuals with life threatening and/or communicable diseases may sometimes be therapeutic or important in the remission or recovery process, or may in some circumstances, even be life sustaining. Co-workers should be sensitive to the needs of an employee with such a condition and recognize that continued employment for an employee suffering from such conditions possibly may be life sustaining and may be both physically and mentally beneficial.

Employee Exposure & Illness

3. An individual with a life threatening and/or communicable illness can continue to work subject to the other rules of the member, so long as he/she is able to continue to perform his/her job satisfactorily, and so long as the best available and current medical evidence indicates that his/her continued employment does not present a direct health or safety threat to himself/herself or others. The qualification that an individual not pose a direct threat to the health or safety to himself/herself or others must apply not just to individuals with life threatening and/or communicable illnesses, but to all applicants and employees.

4. A "direct threat" entails a significant risk of substantial harm. A speculative or remote risk is not sufficient to constitute a direct threat. A determination of whether an individual poses a significant risk of substantial harm to others must be made on a case-by-case basis. The following factors should be considered:

   a. the duration of the risk;
   b. the nature and severity of potential harm;
   c. the likelihood that the potential harm will occur; and
   d. the imminence of the potential harm.

   It is very important that this analysis rely on objective, factual evidence, not on subjective perceptions, irrational fears, personal attitudes, or stereotypes.

5. Even if a direct threat to the health and safety of the individual or others exists, members must consider whether the risk can be eliminated or reduced by making a reasonable accommodation for the individual with a life threatening and/or communicable illness. Once again, this determination must be made on a case-by-case basis. If warranted, reasonable accommodations should be accorded to applicants or employees with life threatening and/or communicable illnesses so long as the accommodations do not pose an undue hardship to the member.

6. All information concerning an employee's medical condition, medical records and history should be kept confidential.

7. Once a member becomes aware that an employee is suffering from a life threatening and/or communicable illness, the employer should ask the employee for a physician's certification as to whether or not he/she is able to continue to work, whether there are limitations upon the work due to the illness or the amount of time needed for recuperation, and whether the employee poses a health or safety risk to himself/herself or others. A member should reserve the right to require an examination of the employee by a physician chosen by the member.

8. In the event a co-worker is concerned about his/her safety and health with regard to working with a colleague suffering from a life threatening and/or

communicable illness, the member should attempt to educate the co-worker with regard to the nature of the illness suffered by his or her colleague, particularly focusing on whether common work place contact with the individual poses a threat of transmission.

9. Employees with life threatening and/or communicable illnesses who are no longer able to work should be treated in a consistent, compassionate manner and offered assistance in managing leave or other benefits.

10. All members should educate their employees about Center for Disease Control (CDC) guidelines and OSHA regulations for the prevention of transmission of life threatening and communicable illnesses in the health care work place. Copies of the applicable CDC guidelines and OSHA regulations should be available at the member's place of business for review by all employees.

11. All members should also be familiar with, and should follow, all applicable federal, state and local laws governing employees with disabilities, medical testing and screening of employees, occupational safety and health, standards of patient care, and confidentiality of medical records.

CASE STUDY

At 1930 hours on a Friday evening, you and your partner are dispatched to a "child seizuring." According to the dispatcher, the child's mother called 911 and stated her child was "convulsing and turning blue."

Upon arrival, you find a three-year-old child who is lethargic, irritable, uncooperative but responds to voice and touch by crying. Vital signs are pulse 120, respirations 36 and noisy. Skin is very warm and flushed. Eyes are reddened, and there is a crusty discharge around the nose.

Mother states the child has had a cold for 2-3 days and had just gotten up from a nap when he began stiffening all over and jerking his arms and head. She states this convulsion lasted a couple of minutes, and he wasn't breathing during the seizure and started to turn blue.

As you initiate a secondary assessment, the child begins seizuring again. You carefully support the child without restraining his activity while your partner begins administering oxygen by face mask. The seizure lasts for approximately 1-2 minutes, and when it stops the child cries weakly.

Because the child feels very warm, you decide to take his temperature which is 104°F (40°C).

After consulting with your medical control doctor, you begin tepid water sponge bath in an attempt to gradually cool the child. Your partner prepares the stretcher, and you place the child in the ambulance. While en route to the hospital the oxygen and sponge bath are continued.

The child is worked up in the emergency department for probable fever unknown origin, URI, R/O meningitis, R/O otitis media, R/O sepsis. He is admitted to the pediatric unit for further evaluation and stabilization of the seizure and temperature.

Two days after admission, your agency is notified by the hospital that the child has been diagnosed with measles. The day after he was admitted he developed a rash over his face and upper trunk that has now spread to the rest of his body. Doctors have learned from the mother that she was unable to complete his vaccine series because they had moved to a new town and had not located a doctor.

Your agency has contacted you and your partner because they were unable to determine what precautions you had taken while caring for the child, nor were they able to determine your immunity status for measles.

While caring for the child you and your partner both wore gloves but no other barriers were utilized. Upon review of your and your partner's health records, it was determined that you had had the measles in 1954, however, your partner had no record of having had the measles or having received measles vaccine.

Q. What action should be taken regarding your partner's immunity status?

A. A measles titer should be drawn on your partner. A titer was drawn and was positive for measles.

Q. After learning the immunity status of your partner what additional actions are required?

A. Both you and your partner have immunity to measles, therefore no further actions are necessary.

Q.. If either of you had been found to have no immunity and therefore were susceptible to measles, what actions would have been necessary?

A. You would have had to remain off work from the 5th through the 21st day after exposure and/or until 7 days after the rash appears.

Q. What additional precautions/barriers were indicated based on patient symptoms?

A. While caring for the child eye and face protection should have been worn to prevent droplets from the child's nose and mouth spraying into the rescuer's mucous membranes.

Ensuring that all prehospital workers are immune to the vaccine preventable childhood diseases reduces the risk that a susceptible worker will be exposed, necessitating loss of work during the incubation and communicable period of the disease. The wearing of appropriate barriers to transmission of droplet or airborne spread diseases, gloves, eye and face protection, will also eliminate or reduce the risk of exposure and infection for susceptible individuals.

CHAPTER FOUR

CLEANING & DISINFECTION

Notes

Care of Contaminated Equipment/Work Areas

DISPOSABLE EQUIPMENT AND SUPPLIES:

Disposable items are to be discarded after single patient use. This includes such items as nasal cannulas, oxygen masks, suction tubes, endotracheal tubes, dressings and bandages and IV equipment. These items should be placed in an appropriate trash bag or container and disposed of in accordance with company policy.

Contaminated articles should be handled with care using Universal Precautions to prevent contamination of employee or clean equipment.

REGULATED WASTES

Regulated waste is defined by OSHA as:

- Any liquid or semi-liquid blood or other potentially infectious material.
- Contaminated items that would release blood or OPIM in a liquid or semi-liquid state if compressed.
- Items caked with dried blood or OPIM and capable of releasing these materials during handling.
- Contaminated sharps.
- Pathological and microbiological wastes.

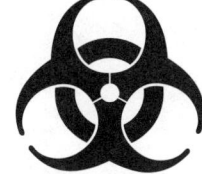
BIOHAZARD

Regulated waste must be placed in a biohazard labelled bag or container and disposed of in accordance with local, state, and/or federal EPA regulations. This often means incinerating the waste or sterilizing prior to hauling to an approved landfill. The container for regulated waste must be closeable, constructed to contain all contents and prevent leakage of fluids, and closed prior to removal to prevent spillage. If the container becomes contaminated, it must be placed in a second container that meets all of the above requirements.

Needles and sharps pose a unique hazard to the HCW and thus require special handling. Needles and/or sharps are not to be broken, bent, sheared, or recapped. An exception to this rule is permitted if there is no feasible alternative and is required for medical reasons. For instance, if a pre-loaded medication syringe is used and only a partial dose is administered and a second dose will be given later necessitating recapping of the syringe. If this occurs, recapping of the needle is permitted, provided the procedure to accomplish this is a one-handed technique or uses a mechanical device to recap the needle.

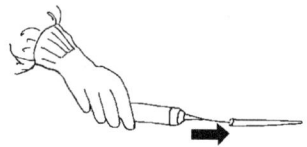

Needles and sharps are to be discarded immediately or as soon as feasible in containers that meet OSHA standards.

Needles and sharps containers must be:

- closeable
- puncture resistant
- leak-proof on sides and bottom
- labelled or color coded as a biohazard
- easily accessible to personnel
- located close to area of use
- maintained in an upright position
- replaced routinely and not allowed to overfill
- closed prior to moving to prevent spillage
- placed in secondary container if leakage is possible

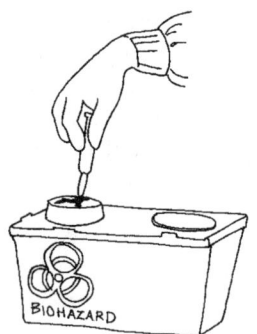

Broken glassware is to be cleaned up using a hands-free technique. A broom and dustpan or other similar procedure may be used.

Cleaning & Disinfection

NON-DISPOSABLE ITEMS AND WORK SURFACES

It is an employer's responsibility to ensure a clean and sanitary work environment for their employees. In addition, equipment used with patients must be cleaned and disinfected and in some cases sterilized between patient uses.

Written schedules for cleaning and methods of decontamination should be developed with these considerations in mind:

- location of area to be cleaned
- type of surface to be cleaned
- type of soil or debris present
- tasks or procedures performed in area or equipment used

Routine cleaning of work and environmental surfaces including cans, bins, pails, shelves, floors and walls of vehicles, benches and seats should be completed on a regular schedule at least once per shift or day. This routine cleaning of surfaces and equipment that has no contact with patients and when no blood or body fluids are present requires the use of an intermediate or low level disinfectant. Follow the manufacturer's recommendations in selection of cleaning and disinfecting solutions and methods for cleaning. Failure to do so can result in damage to surfaces being cleaned.

CDC has developed recommendations for the reprocessing of equipment that is used in the prehospital setting.

For critical equipment, instruments, or devices that penetrate skin or contact normally sterile areas of the body, STERILIZATION is the preferred method of cleaning. Sterilization may be accomplished using steam (autoclave), a gas (ethelene oxide), dry heat or immersion in EPA-approved chemical "sterilant" for 6-10 hours following manufacturer's instructions. Liquids should only be used on those instruments that are impossible to sterilize with heat.

Semi-critical equipment, all reusable instruments or devices that come into contact with mucous membranes requires HIGH LEVEL DISINFECTION. High level disinfecting is accomplished by hot water pasteurization (80-100 C, 30 minutes) or exposure to an EPA-registered "sterilant" chemical for a period of 20-45 minutes per manufacturer's instructions.

Non-critical equipment, instruments, devices, or surfaces that come into contact only with intact skin, and have been contaminated with blood and/or body fluids, need INTERMEDIATE LEVEL DISINFECTANT. An EPA-registered "hospital disinfectant" chemical with a label claim for tuberculocidal activity or commercially available hard-surface germicides or solutions of 1:100 dilution of bleach are effective for this level disinfection, however, choice must be made carefully. The particular item to be cleaned may be adversely affected by the chemical chosen or in some cases may absorb the chemical only to release it later when in contact with a patient. Carefully follow manufacturer's recommendations both of product to be cleaned and the disinfectant to be used.

Remember also to get all instructions and usage information in writing.

LOW LEVEL DISINFECTION is indicated for routine cleaning or removing of soil from non-critical equipment provided there is no blood or body fluid contamination. An EPA-registered "hospital disinfectant" chemical may be used to accomplish this level of cleaning. If blood contamination has occurred, a higher level disinfection is required.

Environmental surfaces such as floors, walls, ambulance benches or seats, and shelves can be cleaned and disinfected using any agent intended for this use.

SPECIAL NOTE: Prior to sterilizing or disinfecting, all visible debris, including blood or body fluids, must be removed. Failure to do so can result in inadequate disinfection, as many disinfectants/sterilants are ineffective (inactivated) in the presence of organic matter.

After thorough cleaning and disinfecting, most patient care products must be thoroughly rinsed to remove all traces of the chemical sterilant or disinfectant.

While carrying out all cleaning and disinfecting, personnel should wear appropriate personal protective equipment to prevent exposure to contaminants, blood and/or body fluids and as protection against the cleaning agent itself. Again it is very important to follow all manufacturer's instructions when using these products. Employers are required to provide training in the use of these chemicals and to post Material Safety Data Sheets (MSDS) on all chemicals used in the work place. It is important that personnel know where these are kept and are familiar with their content.

LINENS/CONTAMINATED CLOTHING

If you are with a service that is permitted to leave linens at your receiving hospital, you will need to follow the hospital's policy for handling dirty laundry. Remember, any laundry contaminated with blood and/or body fluids must be handled following Universal Precautions and using authorized personal protective equipment. These linens should be placed in specially designated laundry containers per hospital policy.

If you are a service responsible for your own laundry, you will need to develop several procedures.

Routine laundry should be placed in a container and returned to the base (facility) for appropriate washing. These linens may be washed in a regular washer using a detergent disinfectant.

Linens and other laundry items (i.e. clothing) which have been contaminated with blood and/or body fluids must be immediately placed in a designated container and may not be sorted or rinsed at the site of use.

A biohazard labelled container is required for contaminated linens if persons other than those trained specifically in how to handle contaminated linens may come into contact with them and if Universal Precautions are not followed for all linens.

If only trained persons, using Universal Precautions and familiar with the company's Exposure Control Plan (ECP) have contact with the linens, an alternative labelling system other than the biohazard label may be used.

Cleaning & Disinfection

Contaminated linens may be washed in a regular washer using detergent disinfectant following manufacturer's instructions. Persons handling these linens should be instructed in the company's ECP and wear appropriate personal protective equipment.

If an employee's uniform becomes contaminated with blood and/or body fluids, it should be changed prior to going out on the next call and should not be permitted to be taken home by the employee. The uniform should be properly laundered before being returned to the employee.

CARE OF CONTAMINATED ARTICLES CHART

All articles contaminated by infective material from patients with known or suspected infectious diseases must be decontaminated or disposed of properly. The following is a chart to provide the health care worker with guidelines to determine the type and extent of cleaning that must be completed to ensure adequate decontamination.

To determine whether or not an article has been contaminated, please refer to the charts describing the precautions to be taken with specific isolation types and the infective material. Please note: patients in respiratory isolation will not necessarily have specific infective material, but rather it must be assumed that anything that has come in contact with the air contaminated by the patient is presumed contaminated and therefore must be completely decontaminated.

CLEANING OF CONTAMINATED ARTICLES

ARTICLE	LEVEL OF DISINFECTION	RECOMMENDED METHOD	TIME FOR CLEANING/ SPECIAL NOTES
Airways	High level	sterilant	
Nasopharyngeal	High level	sterilant	20-45 min MR
Oropharyngeal	High level	sterilant	20-45 min MR
Backboards			
If blood present	Intermediate level	HD/TB	MR
No blood/body fluids	Low level	HD	MR
Bag/Valve/Mask	High level	sterilant	20-45 min MR

CODE:

"sterilant" = EPA registered "sterilant"
HD/TB = EPA registered "Hospital Disinfectant" with label claim of tuberculocidal
HD = EPA registered "Hospital Disinfectant"
MR = Manufacturer's Recommendation

ARTICLE	LEVEL OF DISINFECTION	RECOMMENDED METHOD	TIME FOR CLEANING/ SPECIAL NOTES
Bed pans	High level	sterilant	20-45 min MR
Bite blocks	Dispose		EPA rules may apply
B/P cuffs			
bladder, tubes, manometer	Low level	HD	MR
if blood/body fluids	Intermediate level	HD/TB	20-45 min. MR
cuff	Laundry	Detergent disinfectant	MR
Bulb syringe	Dispose		EPA
Cervical collars			
If blood	Dispose		EPA
No blood	Low level	HD	MR
Cold packs	Dispose		EPA
Combi tubes (PTL)	Sterilize or dispose	sterilant	6-10 hr MR
Cricothyroidotomy kit	Sterilize	sterilant	6-10 hr MR
Dressings, bandages	Dispose		EPA
Drug boxes/container			
metal or plastic			
if blood	Intermediate level	HD/TB	MR
if no blood	Low level	HD	MR
cloth (soft packs)	Laundry	Wash in washer with detergent/disinfectant	MR
Emesis basin	High level or dispose	sterilant	MR 20-45 min.
End Tidal CO2 detector units disposable	Dispose		EPA
Endotracheal tubes	Dispose		EPA

CODE:

"sterilant" = EPA registered "sterilant"
HD/TB = EPA registered "Hospital Disinfectant" with label claim of tuberculocidal
HD = EPA registered "Hospital Disinfectant"
MR = Manufacturer's Recommendation

Cleaning & Disinfection

ARTICLE	LEVEL OF DISINFECTION	RECOMMENDED METHOD	TIME FOR CLEANING/ SPECIAL NOTES
Esophageal obturator airway			
masks	High level	sterilant	20-45 min. MR
tubes	Dispose		EPA
E-stretcher			
blood	Intermediate level	HD/TB	MR
no visible blood	Low level or environmental level	HD	MR
External cardiac compression and resuscitation unit (i.e. Thumper, CardiO2, HLR)			
airway tubing	High level or dispose	sterilant	20-45 min. MR
exterior	Intermediate level	HD/TB	MR
respiratory valves	High level	sterilant	20-45 min. MR
Hot packs	Dispose		EPA
Intravenous fluid			
containers	Dispose		EPA
tubing	Dispose		EPA
Intravenous poles			
If blood	Intermediate level	HD/TB	MR
If no blood	Low level	HD	MR
Laryngoscopes			
blades	High level	sterilant	20-45 min. MR
handles	High level	sterilant	20-45 min. MR
Linens			
blankets, cot covers	Laundry	Detergent disinfectant	MR
pillow cases, sheets	Laundry	Detergent disinfectant	MR
Magill forceps	High level	sterilant	20-45 min. MR

CODE:

"sterilant" = EPA registered "sterilant"
HD/TB = EPA registered "Hospital Disinfectant" with label claim of tuberculocidal
HD = EPA registered "Hospital Disinfectant"
MR = Manufacturer's Recommendation

ARTICLE	LEVEL OF DISINFECTION	RECOMMENDED METHOD	TIME FOR CLEANING/ SPECIAL NOTES
MAST trousers			
If blood	Intermediate level	HD/TB	MR
If no blood	Low level	HD	MR
Monitor*, exterior only and			
if blood	Intermediate level	HD/TB	MR
includes patient cable	Low level	HD	MR
and non-disposable lead wires			
Needles and Syringes			
non-reusable	Dispose	Sharps container	EPA
reusable	Sterilize	sterilant	6-10 hr MR
Other electronic equipment* (i.e., I.V. pumps, Apcors, pulse oximetry units,	*Special precautions with electronic equipment. Choice of cleaning agent and method must follow manufacturer's recommendations. Use of other agents may damage electrical components or pose a hazard to user or patient.		
End Tidal CO2 Detecor units*			
If blood	Intermediate level	HD/TB	MR
If no blood	Low level	HD	MR
Oxygen delivery equipment			
extension tubing	Dispose		EPA
face masks	Dispose		EPA
nasal cannula	Dispose		EPA
Oxygen flow meter	Environmental		Caution - see manufacturer's recommendation to avoid fire hazard or damage to unit
Oxygen humidifiers	Sterilize or dispose	sterilant	6-10 hr MR
Oxygen nebulizers	Sterilize or dispose	sterilant	6-10 hr MR

C o d e :

"sterilant" = EPA registered "sterilant"
HD/TB = EPA registered "Hospital Disinfectant" with label claim of tuberculocidal
HD = EPA registered "Hospital Disinfectant"
MR = Manufacturer's Recommendation

Cleaning & Disinfection

ARTICLE	LEVEL OF DISINFECTION	RECOMMENDED METHOD	TIME FOR CLEANING/ SPECIAL NOTES
Oxygen powered positive pressure breathing device (Robertshaw, demand valve, Elders valve, etc.)			
hose	Varies by product		MR
masks	High level or dispose	sterilant	20-45 min MR
Oxygen regulators	Environmental level	*Caution - see manufacturer's recommendation to avoid fire hazard or damage to unit*	
Oxygen tanks	Environmental level	*Caution - see manufacturer's recommendation to avoid fire hazard or damage to unit*	
Penlights	Dispose		
Pillows	Laundry/dispose	Detergent/disinfectant	EPA
Pocket masks	High level	sterilant	20-45 min MR
PTL tubes (Combi tubes)	Sterilize or dispose	sterilant	6-10 hr MR
Restraints			
cloth	Laundry	Detergent/disinfectant	
leather	Scrub with detergent disinfectant		
If blood	Intermediate level	HD/TB	MR
Resuscitators (bag/valve/masks)	High level	HD/TB	20-45 min MR
Safety pins	Dispose	EPA sharps container	EPA
Sandbags	Intermediate level	HD/TB	MR
Dispose		EPA	
Shears or scissors			
If blood	Intermediate level	HD/TB	MR
If no blood	Low level	HD	MR

CODE:

"sterilant" = EPA registered "sterilant"
HD/TB = EPA registered "Hospital Disinfectant" with label claim of tuberculocidal
HD = EPA registered "Hospital Disinfectant"
MR = Manufacturer's Recommendation

ARTICLE	LEVEL OF DISINFECTION	RECOMMENDED METHOD	TIME FOR CLEANING/ SPECIAL NOTES
Splints			
air, metal, wood			
If blood	Intermediate level	HD/TB	MR
If no blood	Low level	HD	MR
cloth support straps	Laundry	Detergent/disinfectant	MR
Sterile solutions once opened (i.e. eye wash, saline solution for burns, etc.)	Dispose		EPA
Stethescope			
If blood	Intermediate level	HD/TB	MR
If no blood	Low level	HD	MR
Straps	Laundry	Detergent/disinfectant	MR
Stretcher			
If blood	Intermediate level	HD/TB	MR
If no blood	Low level	HD	MR
Stylets	Sterilize or Dispose	sterilant	6-10 hr MR EPA
Suction units			
catheters			
flexible	Dispose		EPA
tonsil tip (yankhauer)			
metal	Sterilize	sterilant	MR
plastic	Dispose		EPA
collection unit			
bag	Dispose		EPA
bottle	High level	sterilant	20-45 min MR
tubing from patient to collection unit	High level or Dispose	sterilant	20-45 min MR EPA
unit or machine exterior	Caution - follow manufacturer's recommendation		
If blood	Intermediate level	HD/TB	MR
If no blood	Low level	HD	MR

CODE:

"sterilant" = EPA registered "sterilant"
HD/TB = EPA registered "Hospital Disinfectant" with label claim of tuberculocidal
HD = EPA registered "Hospital Disinfectant"
MR = Manufacturer's Recommendation

Cleaning & Disinfection

ARTICLE	LEVEL OF DISINFECTION	RECOMMENDED METHOD	TIME FOR CLEANING/ SPECIAL NOTES
Thermometers	Sterilize or dispose	sterilant	6-10 hr MR EPA
Tongue blade	Sterilize or dispose or dispose	sterilant	6-10 hr MR EPA
Urinals	High level or dispose	sterilant	20-45 min MR EPA

For further information on selection of clinical disinfectants refer to the EPA for a listing of registered chemicals by their classification and to APIC guideline for selection and use of disinfectants an article by Dr. William Rutala published in *The American Journal of Infection Control,* April 1990, Volume 18, No. 2.

This article more fully describes the use, advantages and disadvantages of the various chemicals and provides very practical advice on the selection of an appropriate germicide for your operation.

CODE:

"sterilant" = EPA registered "sterilant"
HD/TB = EPA registered "Hospital Disinfectant" with label claim of tuberculocidal
HD = EPA registered "Hospital Disinfectant"
MR = Manufacturer's Recommendation

NOTES

Chapter Five

Exposure Control Plan

"The OSHA Rule"

NOTES

A Summary of the Bloodborne Pathogen Standard

The Department of Labor has published an amendment to the Occupational Safety and Health Act (OSHA) which describes requirements for employers of employees who have occupational exposure to bloodborne pathogens.

Enforcement of this rule rests with federal OSHA or with state OSHA officers in those states with state plans. Federal OSHA applies to most employers except municipal employers. In state plan states, the rule applies to municipal employees as well. A listing of state plan states is included in Figure 5.1. While this chapter is provided as a guide to assist in complying with the rule, the employer must review and be familiar with the standard for requirements which apply to their setting.

BACKGROUND

OSHA issued the bloodborne standard to provide protection to 5.6 million workers and to prevent 200 deaths and 9,200 bloodborne infections annually.

While the risk for occupational transmission of HIV is rare, the lethal nature of the infection requires that every precaution be taken to prevent exposure. Infection with hepatitis B or C from occupational exposure occurs more readily than with HIV.

Employers are required to develop exposure control plans that will eliminate or minimize occupational exposure to bloodborne pathogens.

EXPOSURE CONTROL PLAN

The bloodborne pathogen rule requires employers to establish a written Exposure Control Plan designed to eliminate or minimize employee exposure.

The plan must contain at least the following:

1. Exposure determination which shall contain:

    A. A list of all job classifications in which all employees in those job classifications have occupational exposure;

    B. A list of job classifications in which some employees have occupational exposure and;

    C. A list of tasks and procedures in which occupational exposure occurs and that are performed by employees classified in B.

2. The schedule and method of implementation for:

    A. Methods of compliance

    B. Hepatitis B vaccination and post-exposure evaluation and follow-up

    C. Communications of hazards to employees

    D. Recordkeeping of the standard

3. Procedure for evaluation of circumstances surrounding exposure incidents.

A copy of the Plan must be accessible to employees. The Plan must be reviewed and updated at least annually and whenever necessary to reflect new or changed tasks or procedures or new employee positions with occupational exposure.

METHODS OF COMPLIANCE

UNIVERSAL PRECAUTIONS

Universal precautions shall be observed to prevent contact with blood or other potentially infectious materials (OPIM). When differentiation of body fluids is difficult such as occurs in emergency situations or uncontrolled environments, all body fluids should be considered infectious.

Exposure Control Plan "The OSHA Rule"

ENGINEERING AND WORK PRACTICE CONTROLS

Engineering and work practice controls shall be instituted which eliminate or reduce employee exposure. If occupational exposure still exists after instituting these controls, personal protective equipment shall be used.

Examples of engineering controls and work practice controls that should be included in the prehospital environment include:

- Provision of handwashing facilities which are readily accessible to employees, i.e. in station or garage area, separate from areas where food is prepared, stored, or consumed.

- When handwashing facilities are not feasible, antiseptic towellettes or antiseptic hand cleansers with towels may substitute.

- Handwashing policy that ensures employees wash their hands, and any other skin, with soap and water immediately if contact with blood/body fluids occurs and immediately after removal of personal protective equipment.

- Contaminated needles and other sharps cannot be bent, recapped, or removed unless no other alternative and medically required. Any recapping or removal of needle must be done mechanically or using only one hand. Prohibition on breaking or shearing of needles.

- Reuseable sharps must be placed in puncture resistant container until processed.

- All sharps containers (disposable and reuseable) must be:
  - puncture resistant
  - labelled or color-coded
  - leakproof on sides and bottom
  - must prevent or forbid removal by hand

- Eating, drinking, smoking, applying cosmetics or lip balm, and handling contact lenses are prohibited in work areas where there is a reasonable likelihood of occupational exposure. This includes the patient compartment of the ambulance. The cab of the ambulance can be maintained as a clean area provided:
  - Separating partition between cab and patient compartment is closed at any time occupational exposure may occur.
  - All PPE or contaminated clothing/items are removed prior to entering cab.
  - Hands are washed prior to entering the cab.

- Food and drink shall not be stored in refrigerators, freezers, shelves, cabinets, or on counter tops, or bench tops where blood or OPIM are present.

- Procedures involving blood or OPIM shall be done in a manner to minimize spraying, splashing, aerosolizing, or spattering.

- Mouth suctioning/pipetting is forbidden.

- Containers for blood or OPIM shall be leak proof, labelled or color coded, placed in a second container if outside becomes contaminated, puncture-resistant if applicable.

- Equipment shall be decontaminated prior to shipping or servicing, or if unable to decontaminate, must be appropriately labelled as a biohazard and this information conveyed to person or company receiving to ensure appropriate precautions are taken.

PERSONAL PROTECTIVE EQUIPMENT

The employer is responsible for providing personal protective equipment to all employees where there is occupational exposure. This equipment shall include but is not limited to:

- Gloves, disposable, single-use.

- Gloves, utility, to prevent injuries during extrication or when working in other hazardous environments where broken glass or sharps may be present.

- Gowns or other protective outerwear.

- Face shields or

- Masks and eye protection

- Mouthpieces, resuscitation bags, pocket masks, or other ventilation device.

- Surgical caps or hoods and/or shoe covers or boots when gross contamination can reasonably be anticipated.

It is the employer's responsibility to assure personal protective equipment is:

- provided at no cost to employees;

- appropriate (prevents blood or OPIM from reaching employees' clothing, skin, or mucous membrane);

- used appropriately by employees;

- readily accessible in appropriate sizes, and when necessary alternative products to meet needs of employees with allergies to selected gloves;

- cleaned, laundered and/or disposed of at no cost to employees;

- repaired and replaced at no cost to employee;
- removed immediately or as soon as possible if penetrated by blood or OPIM;
- removed prior to leaving work area.

HOUSEKEEPING

CLEANING

Employers must ensure that the work site is maintained in a clean and sanitary condition. A written schedule for cleaning and method of decontamination shall be developed based upon:

- Location within facility
- Type of surface to be cleaned
- Type of soil present
- Tasks or procedure being performed

The schedule shall include:

- Cleaning and decontamination after contact with blood or OPIM.
- Cleaning after completion of procedures.
- Cleaning immediately or as soon as feasible after blood or OPIM spills.
- Cleaning at end of work shift if surface may be contaminated.
- Cleaning of bins, cans and pails that may become contaminated with blood and OPIM.
- Hands-free picking up of broken glassware.

REGULATED WASTE

Contaminated sharps shall be discarded immediately or as soon as feasible and placed in containers which are:

- Closeable
- Puncture resistant
- Leakproof and color coded

- Labelled or color coded
- Easily accessible and located as close as possible to immediate area where sharps are used
- Maintained upright throughout use
- Replaced routinely and not permitted to over fill
- Closed prior to moving to prevent spillage
- Placed in a secondary container if leakage is possible
- Not opened, emptied or cleaned manually if reuseable

Other regulated waste shall be placed in container which are:

- Closeable
- Contructed to contain all contents and prevent leakage
- Labelled or color coded
- Closed prior to moving
- Placed in secondary container if outside becomes contaminated

Disposal of all regulated waste shall be in accordance with applicable federal, state or local regulations.

LAUNDRY

Contaminated linens shall be:

- Handled as little as possible.
- Bagged at site of use and not sorted or rinsed in location of use.
- Placed and transported in bags or containers that are labelled or color coded.
- Placed in leakproof container if soak-through possible.
- Handled by trained employees wearing appropriate PPE.
- Placed in biohazard labelled containers if shipping off site to a laundry that does not utilize universal precautions.

Exposure Control Plan "The OSHA Rule"

No discussion of HIV or HBV research labs and production facilities is included in this section.

HEPATITIS B VACCINATION AND POST-EXPOSURE EVALUATION AND FOLLOW-UP

Employer shall make available to all employees who have occupational exposure, Hepatitis B vaccine and post-exposure evaluation and follow-up for exposure incidents which includes the following:

- At no cost to employee.

- Make available at reasonable time and place.

- Performed by or under direction of physician or other licensed health care professional.

- Provided in accordance with current U.S. Public Health Service recommendations.

- Lab tests are conducted by an accredited lab and at no cost to employee.

- Health care professional's written opinion of evaluation made available to employee within 15 days of evaluation.

HEPATITIS B VACCINATION shall be given to all employees with occupational exposure:

- After receiving required training and within 10 days of initial assignment to job.

- Unless previously vaccinated.

- Unless antibody positive by lab test.

- Unless contraindicated for medical reasons.

- Unless employee refuses and declination statement is signed (See Figure 5.2).

- Booster shots given if recommended by United States Public Health Service.

POST-EXPOSURE EVALUATIONS AND FOLLOW-UP

When an exposure incident occurs, the employer will make immediately available confidential medical evaluation and follow-up including at least the following:

1. Document route and circumstances surrounding exposure.

2. Identify and test source individual as permitted by law and provide results of testing to employee. Employee will be informed of disclosure laws and regulations regarding identity and infectious status of source individual.

3. Collecting and testing of employee's blood for HBV and HIV status. If employee initially refuses testing but allows blood draw, blood will be held for up to 90 days to allow employee to elect to have test done.

4. Post-exposure prophylaxis when medically indicated following U.S. Public Health Service recommendations.

5. Counseling.

6. Evaluation of reported illnesses.

The employer is required to provide the following information to the Health Care Professional (person selected to provide post-exposure evaluation).

- Copy of the regulation.

- Description of exposed employee job duties as related to exposure incident.

- Documentation of route and circumstances of exposure.

- Results of source individual's blood tests if known.

- All relevant medical records of the employee.

The employer is responsible for obtaining and providing the employee with a copy of evaluating Health Care Professional's written opinion within 15 days of evaluation.

COMMUNICATION OF HAZARDS TO EMPLOYEES

LABELS AND SIGNS

Employers are required to provide warning labels on regulated waste containers, and other containers of blood or OPIM. Labels should be fluorescent orange and orange-red and include biohazard symbol and legend.
Biohazard symbol and legend.
Red bags or red containers may substitute for labels.

TRAINING

Employer shall ensure all employees with occupational exposure have participated in a training program that is:

- at no cost to employees
- during working hours
- provided at the time of initial assignment to tasks where exposure may occur
- offered at least annually thereafter and whenever new tasks are introduced or changes in plan occur
- provided by a person who is knowledgeable in subject matter as it relates to this work place
- appropriate in vocabulary and content to educational, literacy level and language of employees

The training program shall minimally contain:

- accessible copy of standard and
- explanation of contents
- explanation of epidemiology and symptoms of bloodborne disease
- explanation of modes of transmission of BBP
- explanation of Exposure Control Plan and how to obtain a copy
- how to recognize tasks that may cause exposure incident
- explanation, use and limitations, of engineering controls, work practice controls, and personal protective equipment to prevent exposures
- information on type, proper use, location, removal, handling, decontamination, and disposal of PPE
- explanation of the basis for selection of PPE
- information on Hepatitis B vaccine
- information on actions to take and who to notify in case of exposure incident

- information on post-exposure evaluation and follow-up
- explanation of labels and signs
- opportunity for interactive questions and answers with person conducting training

RECORDKEEPING

MEDICAL RECORDS

The employer is required to establish and maintain accurate, confidential medical records for each employee with occupational exposure that includes:

- name, social security number
- employee's Hepatitis B vaccine status including dates received and records relative to employee's ability to receive vaccine, or
- signed declination if applicable
- copy of all results of exams, medical testing, and follow-up as required
- employer's copy of Health Care Professional's written opinion after evaluating exposure incident
- copy of information given to Health Care Professional at time of exposure incident.

These records must be kept for duration of employment plus 30 years.

TRAINING RECORDS

Employers are required to maintain training records that include:

- dates of training sessions
- contents or summary of training session
- names and qualifications of person conducting training and
- names of job titles of all persons attending

These records shall be maintained for three years.

In addition to developing and writing an exposure control plan, an employer will want to do monitoring and surveillance to ensure the plan is working and employees are knowledgeable in its content and application. Records documenting monitoring of the plan should be maintained.

When monitoring identifies areas where the plan is not working or there is non-compliance, an action plan to correct deficiency should be undertaken.

The Exposure Control Plan as described may be a part of the company's larger Infection Control Plan or Health and Safety Program. However, it must be easily identifiable within the larger plan and must be able to stand on its own as a separate document in the event an employee requests a copy for review.

FIGURE 5.1

STATES & TERRITORIES WITH OCCUPATIONAL SAFETY AND HEALTH STATE PLANS

Alaska	New Mexico
Arizona	New York
California	North Carolina
Connecticut	Oregon
Hawaii	Puerto Rico
Indiana	South Carolina
Iowa	Tennessee
Kentucky	Utah
Maryland	Vermont
Michigan	Virginia
Minnesota	Virgin Islands
Nevada	Washington
	Wyoming

FIGURE 5.2

HEPATITIS B VACCINE DECLINATION (MANDATORY)

I understand that due to my occupational exposure to blood or other potentially infectious materials I may be at risk of acquiring Hepatitis B Virus (HBV) infection. I have been given the opportunity to be vaccinated with Hepatitis B vaccine at no charge to myself. However, I decline Hepatitis B vaccination at this time. I understand that by declining this vaccine, I continue to be at risk of acquiring Hepatitis B, a serious disease. If in the future I continue to have occupational exposure to blood or other potentially infectious materials and I want to be vaccinated with Hepatitis B vaccine, I can receive the vaccination service at no charge to me.

_____   _____
Employee Signature   Date

_____   _____
Witness   Date

DEFINITIONS FOR THIS CHAPTER

For purposes of this section, the following shall apply:

Assistant Secretary means the Assistant Secretary of Labor for Occupational Safety and Health or designated representative.

Blood means human blood, human blood components, and products made from human blood.

Bloodborne Pathogens means pathogenic microorganisms that are present in human blood and can cause disease in humans. These pathogens include, but are not limited to, Hepatitis B virus (HBV) and human immunodeficiency virus (HIV).

Clinical Laboratory means a work place where diagnostic or other screening procedures are performed on blood or other potentially infectious materials.

Contaminated means the presence or the reasonably anticipated presence of blood or other potentially infectious materials on an item or surface.

Contaminated Laundry means laundry which has been soiled with blood or other potentially infectious materials or may contain sharps.

Contaminated Sharps means any contaminated object that can penetrate the skin including, but not limited to, needles, scalpels, broken glass, broken capillary tubes, and exposed ends of dental wires.

Decontamination means the use of physical or chemical means to remove, inactivate, or destroy bloodborne pathogens on a surface or item to the point where they are no longer capable of transmitting infectious particles and the surface or item is rendered safe for handling, use, or disposal.

Director means the Director of the National Institute for Occupational Safety and Health, U.S. Department of Health and Human Services, or designated representative.

Engineering Controls means controls (e.g. sharps disposal containers, self-sheathing needles) that isolate or remove the bloodborne pathogens hazard from the work place.

Exposure Incident means a specific eye, mouth, other mucous membrane, non-intact skin, or parenteral contact with blood or other potentially infectious materials that results from the performance of an employee's duties.

Handwashing Facilities means a facility providing an adequate supply of running potable water, soap and single use towels or hot air drying machines.

Licensed Healthcare Professional is a person whose legally permitted scope of practice allows him or her to independently perform the activities required by paragraph (f) Hepatitis B Vaccination and Post-exposure Evaluation and Follow-up.

HBV means hepatitis B virus.

HIV means human immunodeficiency virus.

Occupational Exposure means reasonably anticipated skin, eye, mucous membrane, or parenteral contact with blood or other potentially infectious materials that may result from the performance of an employee's duties.

Other Potentially Infectious Materials means

1. The following human body fluids: semen, synovial fluid, pleural fluid, pericardial fluid, peritoneal fluid, amniotic fluid, saliva in dental procedures, any body fluid that is visibly contaminated with blood, and all body fluids in situations where it is difficult or impossible to differentiate between body fluids;
2. Any unfixed tissue or organ (other than intact skin) from a human (living or dead); and
3. HIV–containing cell or tissue cultures, organ cultures, and HIV- or HBV-containing culture medium or other solutions; and blood, organs, or other tissues from experimental animals infected with HIV or HBV.

Parenteral means piercing mucous membranes or the skin barrier through such events as needlesticks, human bites, cuts, and abrasions.

Personal Protective Equipment is specialized clothing or equipment worn by an employee for protection against a hazard. General work clothes (e.g. uniforms, pants, shirts or blouses) not intended to function as protection against a hazard are not considered to be personal protective equipment.

Production Facility means a facility engaged in industrial-scale, large-volume or high concentration production of HIV or HBV.

Regulated Waste means liquid or semi-liquid blood or other potentially infectious materials; contaminated items that would release blood or other potentially infectious materials in a liquid or semi-liquid state if compressed; items that are caked with dried blood or other potentially infectious materials and are capable of releasing these materials during handling; contaminated sharps; and pathological and microbiological wastes containing blood or other potentially infectious materials.

Research Laboratory means a laboratory producing or using research-laboratory-scale amounts of HIV or HBV. Research laboratories may produce high concentrations of HIV or HBV but not in the volume found in production facilities.

Source Individual means any individual, living or dead, whose blood or other potentially infectious materials may be a source of occupational exposure to the employee. Examples include, but are not limited to, hospital and clinic patients; clients in institutions for the developmentally disabled; trauma victims; clients of drugs and alcohol treatment facilities; residents of hospices and nursing homes; human remains; and individuals who donate or sell blood or blood components.

Sterilize means the use of a physical or chemical procedure to destroy all microbial life including highly resistant bacterial endospores.

Universal Precautions is an approach to infection control. According to the concept of Universal Precautions, all human blood and certain human body fluids are treated as if known to be infectious for HIV or HBV, and other bloodborne pathogens.

Work Practice Controls means controls that reduce the likelihood of exposure by altering the manner in which a task is performed (e.g. prohibiting recapping of needles by a two-handed technique.)

CASE STUDY

The following case study describes an occupational situation that is likely to affect emergency medical and public safety workers.

I. At 03:00 hours you are dispatched to a reported stabbing. You arrive to find a 32-year old male with two stab wounds to the chest. Your partner establishes the IVs while you manage the airway. After the call, at the hospital while cleaning the back of the ambulance, you accidentally stick yourself with the bloody IV needle.

Q. What are the steps that should be followed for a post exposure follow-up?

A.
1. Clean wound.

2. Report the exposure incident to employer who shall make immediately available to the exposed employee a confidential medical evaluation and follow-up.

3. Document the route of exposure and the circumstance(s) under which the exposure occurred.

4. Identify and document the source individual unless identification is unfeasible or prohibited by state or local law.

5. Test the source individual's blood as soon as feasible and after consent is obtained in order to determine HBV and HIV infectivity. If consent is not obtained, the employer shall establish that legally required consent cannot be obtained. When the source individual's consent is not required by law, the source individual's blood, if available, shall be tested and results documented.

6. When the source individual is already known to be infected with HBV or HIV, testing for the source individual's known HBV or HIV status need not be repeated.

7. Results of the source individual's testing shall be made available to the exposed person. The exposed person shall be informed of applicable laws and regulations concerning disclosure of the identity and infectious status of the source individual.

8. The exposed person's blood shall be collected as soon as feasible and tested after consent is obtained.

9. If the exposed person consents to the baseline blood collection, but does not give consent at that time for HIV serologic testing, the sample shall be preserved for at least 90 days.

10. Post exposure prophylaxis when medically indicated as recommended by USPHS.

11. The exposed person shall be offered counseling by a Health Care Professional.

12. The employer will provide: a copy of the final rule on bloodborne pathogen subpart Z of 29 CFR part 1910.1030. A description of the exposed employee's duties as they relate to the exposure incident, documentation of the route of exposure and circumstances under which the exposure occurred. Results of source individual's blood testing if available. All medical records relevant to the appropriate treatment of the employee including vaccination status.

13. A copy of the Health Care Professional's written opinion shall be provided to the exposed person within 15 days of the completion of the evaluation.

14. The employer shall establish and maintain an accurate record including employee's name and social security number, copy of hepatitis B vaccination status including dates of all the hepatitis B vaccinations and any medical record relative to the employee's ability to receive the vaccination. A copy of results of examinations, medical testing and follow-up procedures as required, a copy of the HCP written opinion and information provided to the Health Care Professional. These records shall be kept confidential and maintained for at least the duration of employment plus 30 years.

Chapter Six

Training & Education

Notes

TRAINING

Organizations need to develop a comprehensive infection control training program for their staff. This program should contain at a minimum general information on how communicable diseases are transmitted and how to prevent that transmission; information on common communicable diseases or those of particular concern to their employees; a complete training program in the agency's Exposure Control Plan and Bloodborne Diseases as required by OSHA; training in tuberculosis and its prevention and control, as well as training in the safe use of chemicals used to decontaminate equipment. This latter is a requirement under OSHA's Hazardous Communication rule, more often referred to as the "Right to Know" law.

The following is an outline of an Infection Control Training Program guide. Two sections, the Exposure Control Training and Tuberculosis sections, are more fully developed with information formatted to permit copying and enlarging for overheads.

Detailed information for lecture content of the following can be found in the appropriate sections of this book.

I. GENERAL INFECTION CONTROL

A. INTRODUCTION
1. Definitions
   a. Communicable Disease
   b. Infectious Disease
3. Virus
4. Bacteria
5. Antibody
6. Pathogen
7. Microorganisms

B. HOW ARE DISEASES TRANSMITTED
1. Three Essential Elements
   a. Source
   b. Means of Transmission
   c. Susceptible Host
2. Sources of Infection
   a. Persons
   b. Animals
   c. Inanimate object
   d. Environment
3. Means (Routes of Transmission)
   a. Contact
      - Direct
      - Indirect
      - Droplet
   b. Vehicles
      - Food
      - Water
      - Drugs
      - Blood
   c. Airborne
      Droplet Nuclei
   d. Vectorborne
      Mechanical
      Biological

C. HOW TO PREVENT TRANSMISSION
1. Universal Precautions
2. General Isolation Precautions
3. Barrier Techniques - Personal Protective Equipment
   a. Gloves
      Disposable
      Utility
   b. Masks
   c. Face/shields or mask and eye protection
   d. Gowns - Outwear protection
      Booties
      Head protection

D. COMMON COMMUNICABLE DISEASES
1. Bloodborne Pathogens - see ECP
2. Childhood Diseases
3. Meningitis
4. Pneumonia(s)
5. Diphtheria
6. Polio
7. Tetanus
8. Gastro-intestinal Illnesses
9. Scabies, Lice, Ticks

10. Wound Infections
11. Herpes
12. Upper Respiratory Infections

E. CLEANING AND DECONTAMINATION
1. Cleaning Principles
   a. Mechanical cleaning
   b. Removal of all debris, organic matter
2. Principles of Disinfection
   a. Sterilization
   b. High level disinfection
   c. Intermediate level disinfection
   d. Low level disinfection

F. DISPOSABLE SUPPLIES
1. General Trash
2. Regulated Wastes Handling
   a. Needles and sharps
   b. Other
3. Disposal of Trash
   a. EPA regulations
   b. State, local regulations

G. EMPLOYEE HEALTH PRACTICES
1. General Good Health
2. Good Hygiene
3. Immunizations Recommended
4. Exposure Follow-up
5. Employee Illnesses

II. EXPOSURE CONTROL PLAN TRAINING FOR BLOODBORNE DISEASES

A. OBJECTIVES
1. Upon completion the emergency medical worker will be able to:
   a. Define an exposure incident
   b. Identify how bloodborne pathogens are transmitted
   c. Recognize the definitions of HIV, HBV, AIDS and T.B.
   d. Recognize who is at risk of infection
   e. Identify personal behaviors and practices that reduce risk of HIV, HBV and T.B.
   f. Identify work place situations in which people may encounter HIV, HBV and T.B.
   g. Identify situations in which wearing personal protective equipment (gloves, gowns, eyewear, and mask) is recommended.
   h. Identify recommended PPE devices and methods used for disinfecting.

i. State correct procedures for handwashing, needle handling and disposal, handling of specimens, spills and soiled laundry, cleaning surfaces, disinfecting equipment.
j. Recognize childhood diseases.
k. List the routes of transmission of diseases.
l. List the required elements of an exposure control plan as described by OSHA in the Federal Register, December 6, 1991.
m. Describe the engineering controls, work practice controls, personal protective equipment, housekeeping, laundering and regulated waste management to be incorporated in their exposure control plan per OSHA.
n. Describe the epidemiology, symptoms and modes of transmission of bloodborne diseases as identified by OSHA in the Federal Register, December 6, 1991.
o. Describe the essential elements of a hazard communication program for employees with potential occupational exposure to bloodborne pathogens per OSHA.
p. Describe the elements of a Hepatitis B vaccine and Post-Exposure evaluation and follow-up program for employees at risk for occupational exposure to bloodborne pathogens per OSHA.
q. Describe the penalties that may be assessed employers by OSHA for violations of this regulation.
r. List the recordkeeping requirements for Employee Medical Records and Training Records as described by OSHA in the Federal Register, December 6, 1991.

B. LECTURE OUTLINE
1. Introduction to Bloodborne Pathogens
   a. Definitions
   b. Route of Transmission
      1. High Risk Behavior
      2. Occupational Exposure
   c. Epidemiology
      1. Identification (Signs & symptoms)
      2. Infectious agent
      3. Incidence
      4. Mode of transmission
      5. Incubation period & period of communicability
      6. Preventive measures
   d. Universal Precautions
2. Epidemiology of Bloodborne Diseases
   a. Hepatitis B
   b. AIDs
      1. HIV 1
      2. HIV 2
   c. Non-A, non-B Hepatitis
      1. Hepatitis C
      2. Delta Hepatitis

Training & Education

   d. Other bloodborne diseases
    1. Syphilis
    2. Malaria
    3. Babesiosis
    4. Brucellosis
    5. Leptospirosis
    6. Arboviral infection (Colorado Tick Fever)
    7. Relapsing fever
    8. Creutzfeldt-Jakob
    9. Human T-lymphotropic Virus Type I (HTLV-1)
    10. Viral hemorrhagic fever
     (Lassa, Marburg, Ebola, Crimean-Congo)
  3. Exposure Control Methods
   a. Universal Precautions
   b. Engineering Controls
   c. Work Practice Controls
   d. Personal Protective Equipment
   e. Avoidance of high risk behavior
  4. Summary
  5. Question & Answer Period

C. EPIDEMIOLOGY OF BLOODBORNE PATHOGENS
 1. Introduction
  a. Definitions
   1. AIDS: Acquired Immunodeficiency Syndrome, a severe life-threatening syndrome; the late clinical stage of infection with HIV.
   2. Bloodborne Pathogens: Certain pathogenic microorganisms found in the blood of infected individuals.
   3. Bloodborne diseases: Diseases caused by bloodborne pathogens; may be transmitted from the infected individual to others by blood or certain body fluids.
   4. Communicable disease: A disease that may be transmitted directly or indirectly from one person to another.
   5. Contagious: Communicable, transmitted readily from one person to another.
   6. Exposure incident: Means a specific eye, mouth, other mucous membrane, non-intact skin, or parenteral contact with blood or other potentially infectious materials that results from the performance of an employee's duties.
   7. HIV: Human Immunodeficiency Virus, the cause of AIDS.
   8. HBV: Hepatitis B Virus
   9. Infection: State of condition in which the body or a part of it is invaded by a pathogenic agent (microorganism or virus) that, under favorable conditions, multiplies and produces effects that are injurious.
   10. Infectious disease: Any disease caused by growth of pathogenic microorganisms in the body. May or may not be contagious.

11. Non-intact skin: Skin that is open, cut, chapped, abraded, weeping, or having rashes or eruptions.
12. Pathogen: Disease causing substance.
Additional definitions may be found in the:
Federal Register December 6, 1991 page 64175.
A Curriculum Guide for Public Safety and Emergency Response Workers NIOSH, 1989, Section 6: Glossary

b. Route of Transmission
1. Contact with blood and/or certain body fluids through percutaneous injury, non-intact skin or mucous membrane. Vector-borne (mosquito, tick) transmission has occurred with some bloodborne diseases but not with HIV/AIDS.
2. High Risk Transmission Categories
   a. Homosexual/bisexual males
   b. Intravenous drug abusers
   c. Transfusion recipients (before 1985)
   d. Hemophiliacs/coagulation disorders (before 1985)
   e. Sexual partners of any of the above
   f. Children of infected parents
   g. Multiple sex partners
3. High Risk Behavior
   a. Anal sex with or without a condom
   b. Vaginal or oral sex with someone who has or does use IV drugs or engages in anal sex
   c. Sex with someone you do not know well or with someone who has several sex partners
   d. Unprotected sex with an infected person
   e. Sharing IV drug needles or equipment
4. Occupational Exposures
   a. Needlestick injuries
   b. Injuries from other sharps (broken glass, scalpels)
   c. Blood and/or body fluids touching open wounds, cuts or non-intact skin
   d. Blood and/or body fluids touching mucous membrane of eye, nose or mouth
5. Relative risk of occupational exposure resulting in infection is very small for HIV infection, more so for HBV infection. Studies indicate that the risk of developing HIV infection after a needlestick from a known HIV infected person is about 0.5%. The risk of acquiring HBV infection after a needlestick from a known HBV infected person is between 6-30%.

c. Epidemiology
1. Identification: Clinical findings that lead to a diagnosis of an infectious disease.
2. Infectious Agent: Microorganism that causes the disease.
3. Incidence: Frequency of occurrence of any event or condition over a period of time and in relation to the population in which it occurs. Prevalence.

4. Mode of Transmission: The means by which a disease or disease-causing organisms are transferred from one to another.
5. Incubation Period: Time period between infection and appearance of symptoms.
6. Period of Communicability: Period of time in which an infected person is capable of infecting another individual.
7. Preventive Measures: Recommended prophylactic treatment/measures prior to exposure or at time of exposure.

d. Universal Precautions

All patients should be assumed to be infectious for HIV and other bloodborne pathogens.

Blood and certain body fluids (amniotic fluid, pericardial fluid, pleural fluid, synovial fluid, cerebrospinal fluid, semen and vaginal secretions, breast milk, and body fluid visibly contaminated with blood should be assumed to be infectious for HIV and other bloodborne pathogens.

However, when emergency medical and public safety workers encounter body fluids under uncontrolled, emergency circumstances in which differentiation between fluid types is difficult if not impossible, they should treat all body fluids as potentially hazardous.

Incorporates development of guidelines for engineering controls, work practice controls, and personal protective equipment so as to minimize the risk of acquiring bloodborne pathogens during performance of job duties.

HANDWASHING: Hands and other body surfaces should be washed immediately and thoroughly if contaminated with blood or other body fluids to which universal precautions apply, or potentially contaminated articles. Hands should always be washed after gloves are removed.

D. SPECIFIC BLOODBORNE DISEASES

1. Hepatitis B
    a. Identification: Disease in which the virus infects and replicates in the liver. Infection can result in one of two types of outcome–self-limited, acute hepatitis B or chronic HBV infection.

    Self-limited, acute Hepatitis B: Hepatitis B virus enters the body and attacks and infects the liver. Infection with the virus can be identified by testing for the presence of hepatitis B surface antigen (HBsAg) and/or hepatitis B core antigen (HBcAg) and/or hepatitis B e antigen (HBeAg). As the body responds to the presence of the hepatitis antigens, antibodies are formed. The presence of hepatitis B surface antibodies (Anti-HBs), coincides with the destruction of infected liver cells, elimination of the virus from the body and signifies lifetime immunity to the virus. It is this destruction of liver cells that is responsible for most of the symptoms observed. The onset of symptoms is often insidious.

Severity of symptoms ranges from no symptoms to a very mild flu-like to the most severe that includes jaundice, dark urine, extreme fatigue, anorexia, nausea, abdominal pain, joint pain, rash and fever. These more severe symptoms can result in hospitalization and extended recuperation times. One to two percent of all acute hepatitis B cases will develop fulminant hepatitis which is about 85% fatal. Chronic HBV infection has more severe long term consequences. In this situation the individual does not develop antibodies to the HBsAg and cannot clear the virus from his liver. As a result he becomes a lifelong carrier of the virus. Such persons are at high risk for developing chronic, persistent hepatitis, cirrhosis of the liver and primary liver cancer. Pregnant women who are chronic carriers and test positive for HBeAg at time of delivery are very likely to pass on infection to their newborn.

b. Infectious Agent: hepatitis B virus (HBV)
c. Incidence: Found worldwide in humans; over 5% of adult USA population has anti-HBs indicating previous infection. 0.2-0.9% of USA population is HBsAg positive (carriers). "High risk groups include IV drug abusers, heterosexuals with multiple partners, homosexual men, clients and staff in institutions for the retarded, patients and employees in hemodialysis centers and persons in certain health care and public safety occupations."[1] Studies in these latter groups have found anti-HBs in 10-30% of the population tested.
d. Mode of Transmission: Exposure to blood and/or body fluids via percutaneous needlesticks, perinatal exposure, sexual intercourse, transfusions of unscreened or untreated blood or blood components, contact with non-intact skin or mucous membrane. Household contacts have developed infection after sharing common items such as razors or toothbrushes.
e. Incubation & Period of Communicability: Incubation is usually between 45-180 days, but may be as short as two weeks or as long as 6-9 months. This variation is related to the amount of virus present in the fluid, mode of transmission and host factors. Individuals can be infectious for many weeks prior to onset of symptoms, throughout the acute clinical course and during chronic carrier states. Individual is no longer considered infectious when testing indicates presence of anti-HBs and absence of antigen (HBeAg).
f. Preventive Measures: Two types of vaccine are available. Both have been shown to be safe and highly effective. One is plasma-derived vaccine prepared from plasma of chronic carriers. The second type of vaccine is made by recombinant DNA technology. Both vaccines are given in 3 IM doses initially and 1 and 6 months later. CDC recommends vaccine be given to those individuals at high risk of infection including occupational exposure. OSHA requires employers to provide hepatitis B vaccine at no

charge to all employees at risk for occupational exposure. Recommendations for post-exposure prophylaxis is fully described in the CDC publication, MMWR February 9, 1990, Vol 39, No. RR-22. HBV carriers should be cautioned regarding their need to avoid conditions that put them at risk to transmit the virus to other individuals.

2. Acquired Immunodeficiency Syndrome (AIDS)
   a. Identification: AIDS is the late and usually most severe stage of infection with HIV. Infection begins after exposure to HIV virus. HIV1 and HIV2 are human retroviruses. This means that they cannot replicate except within a living cell. HIV virus invades cells of the immune system in its human host, specifically the macrophages and the T4 lymphocytes or helper cells. As the virus replicate, more and more cells of the immune system become infected and rendered useless, causing the individual to become susceptible to opportunistic infections. Some viruses can be transported through the bloodstream in macrophages and eventually end up in the brain leading to neurological complications. After an exposure, infection with HIV can occur usually within 6-12 weeks. An initial mono-like illness is usually described within two weeks to two months of the exposure. This initial illness is usually self-limiting (1-2 weeks). Infected individuals may then remain symptom free for months to years before other opportunistic diseases, neurological complications or "wasting syndrome" develop. The CDC in fall, 1992, revised the case definition for the diagnosis of AIDS. These conditions include Pneumocystis carinii pneumonia, chronic intestinal cryptosporidiosis or isosporiasis, toxoplasmosis of the brain, esophageal or respiratory tract candidiasis, extrapulmonary cryptococcosis, coccidioidomycosis, disseminated atypical mycobacteriosis, cytomegalovirus (CMV) infection other than liver, spleen or nodes, chronic ulcerative mucocutaneous or disseminated herpes simples infection and progressive multifocal leukoencephalopathy, recurrent salmonella septicemia, disseminated histoplasmosis; cancers include Kaposi's sarcoma, primary B-cell lymphoma limited to the brain and non-Hodgkin's lymphoma, wasting syndrome, extrapulmonary tuberculosis, HIV related encephalopathy, invasive cervical cancer, pulmonary tuberculosis and recurrent pneumonia with evidence of HIV infection. In addition patients with HIV and whose CD4 T cell count is 200 or less are classified as having AIDS. Infection with HIV can be identified by testing the blood for presence of HIV antibodies. Usually the blood is tested using the ELISA technique. This test is very sensitive and economical. The test is negative if no HIV antibodies are present; if the test is positive, a second ELISA test is run on the blood sample. If this second test is positive, a confirmatory test is conducted using the Western Blot technique. This test is more specific but less sensitive than the ELISA and is used to validate the

first test. If both tests are positive, it is indicative of the presence of HIV antibodies and HIV infection. One major disadvantage to antibody testing is that if the individual being tested was recently infected and has not developed antibodies the test will report negative. It is estimated that this window period, when an individual is infected and capable of transmitting HIV virus to others but is antibody negative, may be as long as six months. Newer tests are currently being developed that will test for the presence of virus itself rather than antibodies, thus allowing for earlier detection of disease.

b. Infectious Agent: Human Immunodeficiency Virus Type 1 and Type 2.

c. Incidence: Worldwide in humans; however, largest number of cases are in the USA. Earliest cases (1970s) occurred in the USA, Haiti, Africa and Europe. Has now spread to virtually every country in the world. In 1990 it was estimated that there were one million persons infected with HIV in the U.S. and 6-8 million cases worldwide. HIV-1 is found in most countries, HIV-2 has been found primarily in West Africa and in countries linked epidemiologically with West Africa. The first case of HIV-1 infection was reported in the USA in 1981, and additional cases have been reported since that time.

d. Mode of Transmission: Documented routes of transmission of HIV includes: sexual intercourse, using contaminated IV needles and equipment, having parenteral, mucous membrane or non-intact skin contact with infected blood, blood components or blood products, receiving transplants of infected organs or tissues, or transfusions of infected blood, through semen used for artificial insemination and perinatal transmission (from mother to child around the time of birth). HIV virus is NOT transmitted by casual contact, or by vectorborne (mosquito, tick) means.

e. Incubation & Period of Communicability: Incubation period is variable. The median time for onset of symptoms is eight years with an observed range of from two months to ten years from infection to the diagnosis of AIDS. The period of communicability is unknown but is presumed to begin shortly after infection and extend throughout life.

f. Preventive Measures: There is no vaccine and no cure for AIDS at this time. Prevention depends on avoidance of those activities that put one at risk for acquiring infection and include: sex with someone who is infected or engages in high risk behavior, anal sex, sharing of IV needles or equipment, percutaneous, mucous membrane or non-intact skin exposure to blood and/or body fluids. Occupational exposures can be minimized by strict adherence to UNIVERSAL PRECAUTIONS, with observance of good hand washing procedure, needle and sharp precautions, appropriate use of PPE.

3. Non-A, Non-B Hepatitis
   a. Identification: Similar to Hepatitis B
   b. Infectious Agent: Unknown but probably more than one; diagnosis is made in absence of hepatitis A or hepatitis B virus.
   c. Incidence: Worldwide in humans (See hepatitis C and Delta).
   d. Mode of Transmission: Same as for Hepatitis B.
   e. Incubation & Period of Communicability: Probably similar to Hepatitis B.
   f. Preventive Measures: No vaccine is available. Universal Precautions the same as for Hepatitis B are recommended. CDC considers it reasonable to give immune globulin (IG) as treatment to persons exposed to known non-A, non-B infected blood.
4. Hepatitis C
   a. Identification: Same as for Hepatitis B, with recent development of a test for antibody to hepatitis C, but diagnosis is usually dependent upon elimination of all other causes of disease.
   b. Infectious Agent: Hepatitis C Virus (HCV)
   c. Incidence: Worldwide in humans; most cases are associated with transfusions, and in the USA it accounts for 90% of the post-transfusion hepatitis cases.
   d. Mode of Transmission: Primarily through transfusions of blood but can be transmitted to health care workers through blood exposures the same as for Hepatitis B.
   e. Incubation & Period of Communicability: Incubation is usually 2 weeks to 6 months. It is communicable from one or more weeks prior to appearance of symptoms, throughout the acute clinical course, and indefinitely in carrier states.
   f. Preventive Measures: Same as non-A, non-B hepatitis, no vaccine available.
5. Delta Hepatitis
   a. Identification: Onset is usually abrupt. Signs and symptoms are similar to Hepatitis B and is always coexistent with Hepatitis B infection. Diagnosis is made by testing for antigen and/or antibody.
   b. Infectious Agent: Hepatitis Delta Virus (HDV).
   c. Incidence: Worldwide but prevalence varies widely. Appears in populations at risk for Hepatitis B.
   d. Mode of Transmission: Same as for Hepatitis B.
   e. Incubation & Period of Communicability: Unknown in humans; blood is potentially infectious through all phases of infection.
   f. Preventive Measures: No vaccine and no treatment at this time. Universal Precautions as for Hepatitis B. However, immunity to Hepatitis B ensures protection against Delta Hepatitis.
7. Syphilis
   a. Identification: Following infection and an incubation period, the disease will manifest itself in three stages if untreated. The primary phase is characterized by the appearance of a single lesion (chancre), a painless lesion with serous exudate. Untreated this

lesion will resolve within weeks. The secondary phase begins 4-6 weeks later with the appearance of a symmetrical maculopapular rash on the palms and soles, accompanied by fever and adenopathy. The secondary phase resolves within weeks to 12 months. The majority of patients will then go into a latency period of weeks to years. The third phase or tertiary syphilis is characterized by involvement of many body systems including skin, bones, CNS and cardiovascular system with high morbidity and mortality. Laboratory evidence of the presence of spirochetes may be demonstrated during the initial phase and throughout clinical infection, although it is markedly reduced during tertiary syphilis.

    b. Infectious Agent: Treponema pallidum, a spirochete.
    c. Incidence: Widespread, primarily found in young people (20-35 years). More prevalent in urban areas and in lower socioeconomic areas.
    d. Mode of Transmission: Primarily sexually transmitted or in utero. However, there are documented cases of transmission by needle-stick, by tattooing instruments and by blood transfusions, or on the hands of health care workers after examining infected lesions.
    e. Incubation & Period of Communicability: Incubation period is between 10 days and 3 months. Communicability is variable and indefinite. Effective antibiotic treatment usually ends infectivity within 24-48 hours.
    f. Preventive Measures: No vaccine available. Same precautions as for Hepatitis B. Preventive treatment with an effective antibiotic during the incubation period would be expected to prevent manifestation of symptoms and serological test positivity.

8. Malaria
    a. Identification: Potentially fatal illness characterized by paroxysms of fever, chills, anemia, sweats and may progress to more severe CNS symptoms including coma and other organ failures. Laboratory evidence confirms the presence of malaria parasites in the blood. The disease may manifest in intervals of symptoms occurring every day, every other day or every third day. Duration of illness in untreated persons lasts from a week to a month or longer. The disease is characterized by relapses between periods of no parasitemia. This may continue irregularly for 2 to 5 years and in some cases for up to 50 years.
    b. Infectious Agent: Plasmodium vivax, P. malariae, P. falciparum and P. ovale.
    c. Incidence: No longer a major problem in temperate or affluent tropical environments but does remain a problem in tropical environments where there are low socioeconomic conditions. In the late 1980s there were several outbreaks of mosquito-borne malaria in Southern California.
    d. Mode of Transmission: Mosquito-borne transmission is the primary mode. May also be transmitted through needlesticks or

transfusions or by sharing of IV needles or equipment.
   e. Incubation & Period of Communicability: The time between the infective bite and the appearance of symptoms is variable depending on the organism ranging between 12 days and 10 months or longer. Communicability occurs as long as the organism remains in the blood. The mosquito is infectious for life.
   f. Preventive Measures: Universal Precautions and prophylactic anti-malarial chemotherapy when in endemic areas or exposure.
9. Babesiosis
   a. Identification: A relatively rare but serious and sometimes fatal disease caused by infection with a protozoan parasite. Symptoms include fever, fatigue and anemia lasting days to months. In some cases no symptoms are observed. Infection is confirmed by testing for presence of the parasite and by antibody testing.
   b. Infectious Agent: Babesia microti.
   c. Incidence: Found in USA in areas where host tick may be found. Endemic on Nantucket and other islands in Massachusetts, and Shelter Island, and along Long Island Sound. Cases have been reported in Wisconsin and Connecticut. Cases due to another parasite have been reported in California and Georgia.
   d. Mode of Transmission: Transmitted during the summer from the bite of a nympho tick found on voles and deer mice. The adult tick can be found primarily on deer but has been identified on other mammalian and avian host. Transmission has also occurred from blood transfusion with infected blood.
   e. Incubation & Period of Communicability: Incubation period is from 1 week to 12 months. Not communicable between humans except through blood transfusions.
   f. Preventive Measures: Universal Precautions.
10. Brucellosis
    a. Identification: Bacterial illness characterized by fever, chills, sweating, arthralgia, weakness and general achiness. Confirmed by laboratory isolation of infectious organism from blood or other body tissues.
    b. Infectious Agent: Brucella abortus, B. melitensis, B. suis, and B. canis.
    c. Incidence: Worldwide. Primarily a disease of persons who work with infected animals or their tissues, especially veterinarians, farm workers and abattoir workers. Occasional outbreaks from infected cows, sheep or goats. Annual cases in USA < 100.
    d. Mode of Transmission: Contact with tissues, blood, urine, vaginal discharge, aborted fetuses and especially placentas and by ingestion of raw milk or milk products from infected animals. Airborne transmission has occurred in humans in laboratories and abattoirs. Transmission by blood transfusion has been documented.
    e. Incubation & Period of Communicability: Variable from 5-60 days and longer. Communicability would have to be assumed to

be present as long as organism is in blood. Transmission from person to person is not documented except for one transfusion.
   f. Preventive Measures: Universal Precautions. Avoid consuming milk or dairy products that are untreated and/or unpasteurized.
11. Leptospirosis
   a. Identification: Bacterial infection with fever and sudden onset of headache, chills and severe myalgia. Other symptoms include diphasic fever, meningitis, rash, anemia, hemorrhage into skin and mucous membranes, jaundice, mental confusion/depression and pulmonary symptoms. Some cases are asymptomatic and others are often misdiagnosed. Laboratory confirmation of presence of leptospires from blood.
   b. Infectious Agent: Leptospira interrogans, a spirochete.
   c. Incidence: Worldwide, especially to persons exposed to rivers, lakes or other water where infected animals urinate.
   d. Mode of Transmission: Skin contact (especially non-intact skin or mucous membrane with water, moist soil or vegetation contaminated with urine of infected animals or direct contact with urine or tissues of infected animals. No reported cases of transmission from nosocomial exposure to blood have occurred.
   e. Incubation & Period of Communicability: Incubation period is usually 10 days, ranging from 4-19 days. Leptospires are excreted in urine for one month but have been demonstrated for up to 11 months after acute illness.
   f. Preventive Measures: Universal Precautions. Protective outerwear when exposure to potentially infected water or soil may occur.
12. Arboviral Infection (Colorado Tick Fever)
   a. Identification: An acute febrile illness, characterized by diphasic fever, chills, headache, muscle and back aches, neutropenia, and thrombocytopenia. Moderately severe disease can occasionally lead to encephalitis, myocarditis or bleeding. Laboratory confirmation of virus in blood.
   b. Infectious Agent: Viruses of Colorado Tick Fever.
   c. Incidence: Areas above 5000 feet in western Canada, Washington, Oregon, Idaho, Montana, California, Nevada, Utah, Wyoming, Colorado, New Mexico and South Dakota. Several hundred cases are reported annually in the USA.
   d. Mode of Transmission: From the bite of an infected tick. Ticks are found on small mammals. Transmission by blood transfusion has been documented.
   e. Incubation & Period of Communicability: Incubation is usually 4-5 days. Ticks remain infective for life. Virus can be isolated in blood from 2-16 weeks or more after onset of symptoms.
   f. Preventive Measures: Universal Precautions for blood and/or body fluids and avoid ticks or remove from infected patient. Avoid close contact with small animals in endemic regions.

13. Relapsing Fever
    a. Identification: Rare, systemic spirochetal infection characterized by recurring fevers separated by periods of relative well-being. Transitory petechial rashes are common during initial fever. Fatality rate is 2-10% but may go as high as 50% in epidemic louse-borne infections.
    b. Infectious Agent: Louse-borne disease=Borrelia recurrentis. In tick-borne diseases many different strains of spirochetes have been distinguished.
    c. Incidence: Epidemic louse-borne infection has not been reported in the USA in many years. Tick-borne fever has occasionally occurred in limited areas of western states.
    d. Mode of Transmission: Vector-borne, transmission usually occurs while crushing an infective tick thus contaminating the bite wound or abraded skin. Transmission has also occurred when blood from an infected patient contacted mucous membrane of the nose and eyes of health care workers.
    e. Incubation & Period of Communicability: Incubation is from 5-15 days. Louse becomes infective within 4-5 days after ingestion of blood from an infected person and remains so for life. Infected ticks can remain infective for life and can pass infection on to their progeny.
    f. Preventive Measures: Universal Precautions. Control of lice and ticks.
14. Creutzfeldt-Jakob Disease
    a. Identification: A very rare disease characterized by symptoms of confusion, progressive dementia, variable ataxia, myoclonic jerks, spasticity, wasting and coma. Disease progresses rapidly once symptoms begin with death occurring within 3-12 months. Diagnosis is complicated and requires exclusion of other neurological diseases or causes.
    b. Infectious Agent: Virus.
    c. Incidence: Reported from 50 countries, Rare.
    d. Mode of Transmission: In most cases the mode is unknown. Transmission has been documented from infected corneal transplant, insertion of cortical electrodes that had been used on known C-J patients, infected grafts of human dura mater, and several from injections of growth hormone prepared from human pituitary glands. Others have had history of brain or eye surgery within 2 years, and there is one case of a health care worker who became infected while working in a laboratory where she prepared brain specimens and preparing brain specimens for analysis. Actual means of transmission is not known.
    e. Incubation & Period of Communicability: Incubation is long–from 15 months to more than 20 years in iatrogenic cases. Unknown in most cases. CNS tissues are infectious throughout illness. Other tissues and CSF may be infectious. Infectivity not known. Probably begins before symptoms begin.

f. Preventive Measures: Universal Precautions. Careful and thorough disinfecting of instruments used on these patients.
15. Human T-lymphotropic Virus Type I
    a. Identification: Associated with malignant neoplasm of lymphastic tissue, leukemias and lymphomas of T-cells and with a degenerative neurologic disease known as tropical spastic paraparesis or HTLV-1 related myelopathy.
    b. Infectious Agent: HTLV-1.
    c. Incidence: Endemic in southern Japan, Caribbean and in some parts of Africa but also found in USA primarily in IV drug users.
    d. Mode of Transmission: Mother to child through blood or breast milk, transfusions of blood or blood products, sharing of IV needles or equipment and sexual transmission.
    e. Incubation & Period of Communicability: Unknown.
    f. Preventive Measures: Universal Precautions. No vaccine.
16. Viral Hemorrhagic fever (Lassa, Marburg, Ebola, Crimean-Congo).
    a. Identification: Severe viral illness characterized by fever, sore throat, cough, chest pain, vomiting that can progress to hemorrhage, shock, encephalopathy and death. Diagnosis is made by isolation of virus in blood, urine or throat washings.
    b. Infectious Agent: Lassa virus, Marburg virus, Ebola virus, and Crimean-Congo hemorrhagic fever virus.
    c. Incidence: None of these diseases are indigenous to the USA but may occur in persons who have traveled abroad. Lassa fever in West Africa; Marburg has been recognized in Germany, former Yugoslavia, Uganda and Kenya; Ebola disease in the Sudan, Zaire and other areas in sub-Saharan Africa; Crimean-Congo in western Crimean and other areas of the former USSR, former Yugoslavia, Bulgaria, Iraq, the Arabian Peninsula, Pakistan, western China, tropical Africa and South Africa.
    d. Mode of Transmission: Lassa fever by direct or indirect contact with rodent excreta, direct contact with blood, pharyngeal secretions and urine of infected patients and by sexual contact. Marburg disease by direct contact with infected blood, secretions, organs or semen. Nosocomial infections have been frequent. Ebola virus transmission has also occurred as a result of parenteral contact with contaminated needles and syringes with these cases always being fatal. Transmission through semen has occurred 7 weeks after clinical recovery. Crimean-Congo virus is transmitted by bites from infected ticks, to medical workers after exposure to infected blood or secretions, and has occurred in association with butchering infected animals.
    e. Incubation & Period of Communicability: Lassa fever incubation is usually 6-21 days. Persons are communicable while virus can be isolated in their throat, and virus has been isolated in urine up to 9 weeks after onset of illness. Marburg virus incubation is 3-9 days, and Ebola virus incubation is 2-21 days. Communicable as long as virus can be found in blood and secretions. Ebola virus

Training & Education

has been demonstrated in semen up to the 61st day after onset of illness. Crimean-Congo virus incubation is 3-12 days. Tick probably remains infective for life.

    f. Preventive Measures: No vaccines available. Strict adherence to Universal Precautions with all patients blood and body fluids, secretions and excretions. Careful cleaning and decontamination of all items prior to disposal or returned for reuse.

E. EXPOSURE CONTROL METHODS

1. Universal Precautions are to be applied to all patients and to all blood and/or certain body fluids. In emergency conditions where distinction of body fluids is difficult or impossible, all fluids are to be treated as if infectious. Universal precautions include developing and implementing engineering controls and work practice controls that minimize risk of exposures and the use of personal protective equipment when engineering and work practice controls cannot eliminate risk of exposure. Scrupulous hand washing after caring for patients, after cleaning and decontaminating, after removal of gloves and immediately after any exposure to blood and/or body fluids is mandatory.

2. Engineering Controls are considered essential, as they serve to prevent exposures from occurring. Examples of feasible engineering controls are the use of puncture-resistant sharps containers, needleless IV line connectors (stopcocks), and the use of needles with resheathing or retracting devices.

3. Work Practice controls include such things as hand washing policies, use of Universal Precautions, development of written SOPs, policy and communicating hazards to employees and training of personnel in elements of the exposure control plan and SOPs are essential activities.

4. Personal Protective Equipment should be selected that best meets the need to protect employees from occupational exposure to blood and/or body fluids in their work environment. Included in this equipment:
   - disposable gloves (variety of sizes and types)
   - utility gloves to protect workers' hands from sharps during extrication or while providing care in hostile environment
   - face mask and glasses or goggles or the use of a face shield to protect employees' mouth, nose and eyes from splashing or spraying
   - gowns, aprons, or some form of outerwear to protect contamination of clothing and exposed skin
   - booties or head coverings for those conditions involving major trauma and blood and/or body fluids and contamination of shoes or head could reasonably be anticipated
   - resuscitation equipment such as ambubags or pocket masks are useful to prevent the need for direct mouth-to-mouth resuscitation

5. Hepatitis B vaccination program. All employees whose job duties put them at risk for occupational exposure to blood and/or body fluids must be offered Hepatitis B vaccine at no cost to the employee and at a time and place reasonably convenient. Vaccine must be offered within 10 days of initial assignment and after completion of a training program.
6. Avoidance of High Risk Behavior. In addition to training in recognition of occupational exposures and measures to prevent that exposure, training should include information on avoidance of high risk behavior in personal lives. High risk behavior includes:
    - Sex with an infected person or a person who engages in high risk behavior
    - Anal sex
    - Sex with multiple partners or with someone who has multiple partners
    - Sharing of IV needles or equipment

III. EPIDEMIOLOGY OF TUBERCULOSIS AND TUBERCULOSIS INFECTION

A. INTRODUCTION

OSHA has recognized that employees in health care settings are at risk for transmission of tuberculosis. Several recent outbreaks of tuberculosis in health-care settings, including outbreaks involving multi-drug resistant strains of Mycobacterium Tuberculosis, have heightened concern. Transmission of tuberculosis to persons with HIV infections is of particular concern, because they are at high risk of developing active tuberculosis if infected.

B. DEFINITION

Tuberculosis is an acute or chronic infection caused by M. Tuberculosis. It is spread by the airborne route (droplet nuclei) and can spread throughout a room or building carried on air currents. Infection occurs when a susceptible person inhales these droplet nuclei containing T.B. bacilli.

In most individuals, the immune system limits the multiplication and spread of the bacilli in the body, however, some newly infected persons (<1%) will rapidly progress to clinical illness. 5-10% will develop clinical illness months, years or decades after exposure. The risk for developing active disease is increased in individuals with impaired immune systems or those in debilitated condition.

Factors that may enhance transmission include contact between susceptible and infected persons in relatively small, enclosed spaces, inadequate ventilation, re-circulation of air containing droplet nuclei, providing care before diagnosis, performing procedures that cause patients to cough (suction, intubation, aerosol treatments) or patients coughing as a result of clinical condition.

The following recommendations are taken directly from the *Guidelines for Preventing the Transmission of Tuberculosis in Health Care Settings, With Special Focus on HIV-Related Issues.* MMWR, December 7, 1990.

EMERGENCY MEDICAL SERVICES
"When emergency-medical-response personnel or others must transport patients with confirmed or suspected active tuberculosis, a mask or valveless PR should be fitted on the patient. If this is not possible, the worker should wear a PR. If feasible, the rear windows of the vehicle should be kept open, and the heating and air conditioning system set on a non-recirculating cycle.

Emergency-response personnel should be routinely screened for tuberculosis at regular intervals. They should also be included in the follow-up of contacts of a patient with infectious tuberculosis." page 24

C. EPIDEMIOLOGY OF TUBERCULOSIS IN THE UNITED STATES
SUMMARY

Tuberculosis continues to be a public health problem in the United States with over 20,000 cases reported annually. Since 1984 we have not seen the decline in morbidity expected. In fact, there have been substantial increases in tuberculosis morbidity in areas with a high prevalence of human immunodeficiency virus (HIV) infection. In addition to persons with HIV infection, persons at particularly high risk of developing tuberculosis include close contacts of known infectious tuberculosis cases, persons with other medical risk factors known to substantially increase the risk of tuberculosis once infection has occurred; foreign-born persons from high prevalence countries (e.g., those from Asia, Africa, and Latin America); medically underserved low-income populations, including high-risk minorities, especially, Blacks, Hispanics, and Native Americans; alcoholics and intravenous drug users; and residents of long-term care facilities, such as correctional institutions and nursing homes.

D. TRANSMISSION AND PATHOGENESIS
SUMMARY

Tuberculosis is spread primarily be airborne droplets ("droplet nuclei") coughed up by a person with untreated tuberculosis of the lungs or larynx. Close contacts to a person with undiagnosed or untreated pulmonary tuberculosis are at high risk of acquiring infection. About 10 percent of infected persons will develop clinically active tuberculosis at some time in their lives, although the risk is considerably higher in persons who are immunosuppressed. Individuals who are infected but do not have clinically active pulmonary or laryngeal disease are normally not infectious. Transmission of infection can be reduced by: (1) effective chemotherapy of the source case, (2) source case covering mouth and nose when coughing, laughing, sneezing, etc., (3) adequate ventilation, and (4) ultraviolet lights.

- The etiologic agent of tuberculosis, Mycobacterium tuberculosis, is carried through the air in infectious droplet nuclei (small airborne particles less that 5 microns in size) which are produced when persons with tuberculosis of the lung or larynx sneeze, cough, speak, or sing. Infectiousness varies considerably from case to case, e.g. smear positive patients are much more likely to be infectious than smear negative patients and persons with cavitary disease are more likely to be infectious than those without.

- When persons repeatedly breathe air contaminated by an infectious patient, they may become infected with the tubercle bacillus. Normally, persons at highest risk of acquiring infection with tubercle bacilli are close contacts, those living in the same household with the infectious case, or close friends or fellow workers who daily breathe the potentially infectious air from a person with undiagnosed or untreated pulmonary tuberculosis. Infection rates have been relatively stable over the past 12 years, with approximately 29 percent of the close contacts and 15 percent of the other-than-close contacts found to be infected.
- Techniques that reduce the number of airborne droplet nuclei are effective in preventing the transmission of tuberculosis. Covering of the patient's mouth and nose with tissues when coughing or sneezing will reduce the number of organisms excreted into the air. Ventilation with fresh air is important and five or six room air changes per hour are desirable. The number of viable organisms in the air can also be reduced by ultraviolet irradiation of air in the upper part of the room. Masks are of limited value.
- The best way to stop transmission is to start effective anti-tuberculosis therapy which quickly eliminates a large number of a patient's bacilli and renders the patient non-infectious.
- In some individuals exposed to tuberculosis, tubercle bacilli enter the alveoli and establish an infection. Within weeks after the initial infection, tubercle bacilli are spread through the lymphatic channels to regional lymph nodes and then through the blood stream to more distant tissues and organ sites. The tuberculin skin test is used to identify persons who have been infected with the tubercle bacilli. A significant skin test reaction can normally be detected within 2-10 weeks of infection. Individuals who are infected with M. tuberculosis are normally not infectious to others if they have no evidence of clinically active pulmonary or laryngeal disease.
- An average of 1 in 10 infected persons develops the disease at some time in their life unless given preventive therapy. However, persons who are infected with the tubercle bacillus and are immunosuppressed (e.g. those with coexisting HIV infection) are at considerably greater risk of developing clinically active disease. Although the risk of clinical disease is greatest in the first year after infection, disease may occur many years later.
- The lungs are most common sites for clinical tuberculosis. However, tuberculosis is a systemic disease and may also occur as a pleural effusion, miliary disease (disseminated tuberculosis), the lymphatic or

genitourinary systems, or in any other body organ or tissue. In persons with HIV infection, tuberculosis frequently involves extrapulmonary sites; lymphatic tuberculosis and miliary disease are particularly common.

E. SCREENING FOR TUBERCULOUS INFECTION

SUMMARY

Screening for tuberculosis in most U.S. populations is done to identify infected persons at high risk of disease who would benefit from preventive therapy. Screening should be done in groups that experience disease and infection rates substantially in excess of that of the general population. Institutional screening is recommended for staff of acute health care facilities and residents of long-term care institutions where tuberculosis cases are found or the population served has a high incidence of tuberculosis and tuberculous infection. The Mantoux method of administering the tuberculin test is preferred over multiple puncture devices. A reaction of 5 mm is classified as positive in persons who are in close contacts of infectious cases of tuberculosis, those with chest radiographs with fibrotic lesions likely to represent old healed tuberculosis, and persons with HIV infection. A reaction of 10mm is classified as positive in persons not meeting the above criteria, but who have other risk factors for tuberculosis. A reaction of 15 mm is classified as positive in all other persons. A history of vaccination with BCG does not alter the guidelines for the interpretation of the tuberculin skin test in most situations.

TUBERCULIN SKIN TESTING

1. Administration of the tuberculin test

   - Tuberculin skin testing is the standard method if identifying persons infected with M. tuberculosis. The intradermal Mantoux test–not a multiple puncture test–should be used to determine if tuberculous infection has occurred.
   - The Mantoux test is performed by the intradermal injection of 0.1 ml of PPD tuberculin containing 5 TU (tuberculin units) into either the volar or dorsal surface of the forearm. The injection should be made with a disposable tuberculin syringe. The injection should be made just beneath the surface of the skin, with the needle bevel facing upward to produce a discrete, pale elevation of the skin (a wheal) 6mm to 10mm in diameter.
   - To prevent needlestick injuries, needles should not be recapped, purposely bent or broken by hand, removed from disposable syringes, or otherwise manipulated by hand. After they are used, disposable needles and syringes should be placed in puncture-resistant containers for disposal.
   - The Mantoux test should be read 48 to 72 hours after the injection. However, if the patient fails to show up for the scheduled reading, positive reactions may still be measurable up to one week after testing. The reading should be based on measurement

of induration, not erythema. The diameter of induraton should be measured transversely to the long axis of the forearm and recorded in millimeters.
2. Classification of the tuberculin reaction
   - A tuberculin reaction of 5mm or more is classified as positive in the following groups:
   - persons who have had close recent contact with a patient with infectious tuberculosis
   - persons who have chest radiographs with fibrotic lesions likely to represent old healed tuberculosis
   - persons with known or suspected HIV infection
   - A tuberculin reaction of 10mm or more is classified as positive in persons who do not meet the above criteria but who have other risk factors for tuberculosis. This would include:
   - persons with other medical risk factors known to substantially increase the risk of tuberculosis once infection has occurred.
   - foreign-born persons from high prevalence (e.g. those from Asia, Africa and Latin America)
   - medically underserved, low-income populations, including high risk minorities; especially Blacks, Hispanics and Native Americans
   - intravenous drug users
   - residents of long-term care facilities, such as correctional institutions and nursing homes
   - other populations which have been identified locally as having an increased prevalence of tuberculosis
   - A tuberculin reaction of 15mm or more is classified as positive in all other persons.
   - Absence of a reaction to the tuberculin test does not exclude the diagnosis of tuberculosis or tuberculosis infection. Cell-mediated responses such as tuberculin reactions may decrease or disappear during any severe or febrile illness, measles or other exanthemas, HIV infection, live-virus vaccination, Hodgkin's disease, sarcoidosis, overwhelming miliary or pulmonary tuberculosis, and after the administration of corticosteroids or immunosuppressive drugs. Up to 30% of patients without HIV infection and 60% of patients with AIDS may have skin test reactions less than 5mm even though they are infected with tubercle bacilli. In addition, persons who have been very recently infected may not yet have a reaction to the tuberculin skin test.
3. Addressing the "booster" phenomenon
   - The tuberculin skin test can be especially valuable when repeated periodically in surveillance of tuberculin-negative persons likely to be exposed to tuberculosis. However, a problem in identifying newly infected persons is the so-called "booster" phenomenon.
   - Repeated testing of uninfected persons does not sensitize them to tuberculin. However, delayed hypersensitivity to tuberculin, once it has been established by infection with any species of mycobacteria or by BCG vaccination, may gradually wane over the years

in some individuals. When skin tested at this point, these persons may have reactions that are negative. The stimulus of this skin test may recall the hypersensitivity, which results in an increase in the size of the reaction to a subsequent test (a "boosted" response), sometimes causing an apparent conversion interpreted as indicating new infection. Although the booster phenomenon may occur at any age, boosting increases with age and is most frequently encountered among persons over 55. The booster effect can be seen on a second test done as soon as a week after the initial stimulating test and can persist for a year and perhaps longer.

When tuberculin skin testing of adults is to be repeated periodically, the initial use of a two-step testing procedure can reduce the likelihood of interpreting a boosted reaction as representing recent infection. If the reaction to the first test is classified as negative, a second test should be given a week later. If the reaction to the second of the initial two tests is positive, this probably represents a boosted reaction. Based on this second test result, the person should be classified as being infected and managed accordingly. If the second test result remains negative, the person is classified as being un-infected. a positive reaction to a third test (>10mm increase for those less than 35 years old; > 15mm increase for those age 35 years and older) in such a person, within the next two years, is likely to represent the occurrence of infection with M. tuberculosis in the interval (skin test conversion).

4. Interpretation of the tuberculin test in persons with a history of BCG vaccination
   - Many foreign countries still use BCG as part of their tuberculosis control programs, especially for infants. PPD sensitivity and immunity to tuberculosis infection after BCG vaccination is highly variable, depending upon the strain of BCG used and the population vaccinated, so there is no reliable method of distinguishing tuberculin reaction caused by BCG from those caused by natural infections.
   - Positive tuberculin reactions in BCG-vaccinated persons usually indicate infection with M. tuberculosis. Such persons should be evaluated for isoniazid preventive therapy.

F. PREVENTIVE THERAPY TREATMENT OF TUBERCULOSIS INFECTION

SUMMARY

Preventive therapy substantially reduces the risk of developing clinically active tuberculosis in infected persons. Certain groups within the infected population are at greater risk of developing tuberculosis than others. Persons in these groups (e.g. close contacts), should be considered candidates for preventive therapy, regardless of age. The current preventive therapy regimen is six to twelve months of daily isoniazid (10 mg/kg up to 300 mg/day). Patients must be monitored monthly (or more frequently, if necessary) for symptoms of toxicity, as well as to ensure compliance. New, shorter-course preventive therapy regimens are currently being evaluated.

CANDIDATES FOR PREVENTIVE THERAPY

- Skin-test positive persons in the following high-risk groups should be considered candidates for preventive therapy, regardless of age, if they have a positive tuberculin skin test reaction and have not previously been treated:
  1. Persons with known or suspected HIV infection (> 5mm)*
  2. Close contacts of newly diagnosed infectious tuberculosis cases (> 5mm)
  3. Recent tuberculin skin test converters (> 10mm increase within a 2-year period for those less than 35 years old; > 15mm increase for those age 35 years and older).
  4. Previously untreated or inadequately treated persons with chest radiographs showing fibrotic lesions compatible with old healed tuberculosis (> 5mm)
  5. Intravenous drug users (> 10mm)
  6. Persons with medical conditions which have been reported to increase the risk of tuberculosis (> 10mm) (See Section IV, Page 12)

- In addition, infected persons less than 35 years of age in the following high-risk groups are appropriate candidates for preventive therapy, if their reaction to a tuberculin skin test is > 10mm:
  1. Foreign-born persons from high prevalence countries
  2. Medically underserved, low-income populations, including high-risk minorities, especially Blacks, Hispanics, and Native Americans
  3. Residents of long-term care facilities, such as correctional institutions and nursing homes

- Infected persons less than 35 years of age with no additional risk factors for tuberculosis should be evaluated for preventive therapy if their reaction to a tuberculin test is > 15mm. This group should be given a lower priority for prevention efforts than the groups listed above.

- Persons who are close contacts of infectious cases, especially children, should be given preventive therapy regardless of their skin test reaction. After 3 months of preventive therapy, those who were initially skin-test negative should have the tuberculin skin test repeated. Therapy may be discontinued if the skin test is again negative and contact with the infectious case of tuberculosis has been broken.

- For pregnant women who are found to be tuberculin positive upon routine screening, preventive therapy should be delayed until after delivery. However, for pregnant women likely to have been recently infected, isoniazid preventive therapy should begin when the infection is documented, but after the first trimester.

PREVENTIVE THERAPY REGIMEN

- Clinical trials have shown that daily isoniazid preventive therapy for 12 months will reduce the risk of developing tuberculosis in infected persons by about 70 percent and in over 90 percent of patients who are compliant in taking the medication. There is evidence that 6 months of preventive therapy with isoniazid also confers a high degree of protection against the progression to clinically active tuberculosis (approximately 65 percent). Every effort should be made to ensure compliance with preventive therapy for at least six months.
- Twelve months of preventive therapy with isoniazid are recommended for persons infected with tuberculosis who have abnormal chest radiographs (consistent with past tuberculosis) and for persons with HIV infection.
- Isoniazid is normally used alone for preventive therapy in a single daily dose of 10 mg/kg body weight, not to exceed 300 mg per day.
- Isoniazid can also be given twice weekly in a dose of 15 mg/kg (up to 900 mg) when therapy must be directly observed and resources are inadequate to administer therapy on a daily basis.
- Close contacts of infectious tuberculosis patients excreting isoniazid-resistant organisms should be considered for preventive therapy with rifampin (600 mg daily for one year).
- New shorter course preventive therapy regimens (e.g. rifampin and pyrazinamide for 2 months and rifampin alone for 4 months) are currently being evaluated.

MONITORING

- Before preventive therapy is started, it is important to:
- exclude the possibility of current tuberculosis which would require multiple drug therapy;
- question for a history of previous completion of preventive therapy;
- check for contraindications including: previous isoniazid-associated hepatic injury; history of severe adverse reactions to isoniazid, such as a drug fever or rash; acute or active liver disease of any etiology.
- identify patients who need special precautions which include:
  age greater than 35 years; concurrent use of any other medication on a long-term basis (in view of possible drug interactions); daily use of alcohol (which may be associated with a higher incidence of isoniazid-associated hepatitis); possibility of chronic liver disease; existence of peripheral neuropathy or of a condition such as diabetes mellitus or alcoholism (which might predispose to the development of neuropathy); and pregnancy.

- Individuals on preventive therapy should be monitored by questioning for:
- compliance with the prescribed regimen;
- symptoms of neurotoxicity such as paresthesias of hands or feet;
- signs consistent with liver damage such as loss of appetite, nausea, vomiting, persistent dark urine, yellowish skin, malaise, or unexplained elevated temperature of greater than three-days duration, abdominal tenderness (especially right upper quadrant).
- other signs and symptoms the patient may report.
- Patients should be advised to report immediately to their health care provider if any of the above listed or other signs or symptoms occur while taking preventive therapy.
- About 10 to 20 percent of individuals receiving isoniazid will develop some mild abnormality of liver function tests. Because of higher risk for hepatotoxicity among persons over 35 years of age, such persons should have a transaminase test (ALT or AST) at the start of, and periodically, during the course of therapy. If any of these tests exceed three to five times the upper limit of the normal range for that laboratory, the decision to continue isoniazid should be reconsidered. Routine liver function tests are not recommended for persons under the age of 35 years.
- No more than a one-month supply of medicine should be dispensed at a time.
- Monitoring for compliance is especially important for persons on preventive therapy, because they do not have symptoms related to their infection.

G. DIAGNOSIS OF DISEASE
SUMMARY

Pulmonary tuberculosis should be suspected in persons with a productive, prolonged cough (over 3 weeks duration), fever, chills, night sweats, east fatigability, loss of appetite, weight loss, and hemoptysis. The history of exposure to tuberculosis and of previous tuberculosis infection or clinically active disease should be elicited whenever the diagnosis of tuberculosis is entertained. Persons with suspected tuberculosis should be referred for an appropriate examination which should normally include: a history, a histologic examination, a positive bacteriologic culture for M. tuberculosis is essential to confirm the diagnosis of tuberculosis. The chest radiograph may be helpful in making the diagnosis but is never diagnostic for tuberculosis. Initial reports of positive smears or cultures should be reported within 24 hours by telephone to the health department so that a contact investigation can be initiated as quickly as possible.

H. TREATMENT OF DISEASE
SUMMARY

Tuberculosis (disease) should always be treated with at least two drugs. The preferred treatment regimen is of 6-months duration and includes 2 months of daily isoniazid, rifampin, and pyrazainamide, followed by 4 months of daily or twice-weekly isoniazid and rifampin. The 9-month treatment regimen is also acceptable and includes 1 or 2 months of daily isoniazid and rifampin, followed by daily or twice-weekly isoniazid and rifampin, for a total duration of 9 months. Both of these regimens should be supplemented with either ethambutol or streptomycin when isoniazid resistance is suspected or if extensive or life-threatening disease is present. After the initial phase of daily therapy, intermittent therapy (twice weekly) is an effective alternative therapy. Non-compliance with therapy is a major problem in tuberculosis control. Patients must be monitored at least monthly for compliance and adverse reactions to medications.

MONITORING FOR TOXICITY AND RESPONSE TO THERAPY
1. Monitoring for drug toxicity
   Although drug toxicity from anti-tubercuosis drugs is relatively uncommon, it may occur. The health care provider who treats tuberculosis should be familiar with monitoring for toxicity and for response to treatment. For treatment of cases with complications (e.g. drug-resistance, pregnancy, co-infection with HIV, etc.) expert consultation may be required.
2. Monitoring response to treatment
   The best way to measure the effectiveness of therapy for pulmonary tuberculosis is to monitor patients bacteriologically through sputum examination at least monthly until conversion to negative. Patients being treated for uncomplicated pulmonary tuberculosis do not require frequent chest radiographs. Bacteriologic examination is far more important than monitoring chest films.

I. INFECTION CONTROL
SUMMARY

Transmission of tuberculosis infection can be reduced by: effective chemotherapy of the source case; source case covering mouth and nose when coughing, laughing, sneezing, etc.; adequate ventilation; and ultraviolet lights. Precautions to prevent airborne transmission are particularly important during and immediately following procedures which stimulate coughing, e.g. sputum collection, bronchoscopy, and aerosolized pentamidine treatments. Such procedures should be carried out in rooms designated for these procedures with appropriate ventilation.

J. COMMUNITY TUBERCULOSIS CONTROL
SUMMARY

All new tuberculosis cases and suspect cases should be reported promptly to the health department by the health care provider. Early reporting is essential for prompt evaluation of contacts to the source case. Contact investigations (performed by the health department) start with the close contacts who are most likely to be infected. Highest priority is placed on the examination of households where contacts of infectious cases include children.

K. BCG VACCINATION
SUMMARY

BCG vaccination is not normally recommended in the U.S. because of the low risk of infection and the variable effectiveness of the BCG vaccine. A history of vaccination with BCG does not alter the guidelines for the interpretation of the tuberculin skin test in most situations.

Taken from the Core Curriculum on Tuberculosis. Division of Tuberculosis Elimination, Center for Prevention Services, Centers for Disease Control, Atlanta, Georgia and the American Thoracic Society, New York, New York. second edition, April, 1991. United States DHHS, PHS, CDC.~

FIGURE 6.1

OUTLINE OF FINAL RULE ON BLOODBORNE PATHOGENS

SUBPART Z OF 29 CFR PART 1910.1030

a. Scope and Application

b. Definitions

c. Exposure Control
   1. Exposure Control Plan
   2. Exposure Determination

d. Methods of Compliance
   1. General
   2. Engineering and Work Practice Controls
   3. Personal Protective Equipment
   4. Housekeeping

e. HIV and HBV Research Laboratories and Production Facilities

f. Hepatitis B Vaccination and Post Exposure Evaluation and Follow-up
   1. General
   2. Hepatitis B Vaccine
   3. Post Exposure Evaluation and Follow-up
   4. Information Provided to the Health care Professional
   5. Health care Professional's Written Opinion
   6. Medical Recordkeeping

g. Communication of Hazards to Employees
   1. Labels and signs
   2. Information and Training

h. Recordkeeping
   1. Medical Records
   2. Training Records
   3. Availability
   4. Transfer of Records

i. Dates
   1. Effective Date
   2. Exposure Control Plan
   3. Information, Training and Recordkeeping
   4. All Other Provisions

Appendix A: Hepatitis B Vaccination Declination Form

NOTES

TABLE 6.1
RECOMMENDED DRUGS FOR THE INITIAL TREATMENT OF TUBERCULOSIS IN CHILDREN AND ADULTS

Drug	Dosage Forms		DAILY DOSE		MAXIMUM DAILY DOSE IN Children and Adults	TWICE WEEKLY DOSE		Adverse Reactions
			Children	Adults		Children	Adults	
Isoniazid	Tablets:	100 mg*,**, 300 mg	10-20 mg/kg PO or IM	5 mg/kg PO or IM	300 mg	20-40 mg/kg Max. 900 mg	15 mg/kg Max. 900 mg	Hepatic enzyme elevation, peripheral neuropathy, hepatitis hypersensitivity
	Syrup:	50 mg/5 ml						
	Vials:	1 gm						
Rifampin	Capsules:	150 mg*,**, 300 mg	10-20 mg/kg PO	10 mg/kg PO	600 mg	10-20 mg/kg Max. 600 mg	10 mg/kg Max. 600 mg	Orange discoloration of secretions and urine; nausea, vomiting, hepatitis, febrile reaction, purpura (rare)
	Syrup: Formulated from capsules,	50 mg/5 ml						
	Vials:	600 mg						
Pyrazinamide	Tablets:	500 mg**	15-30 mg/kg PO	15-30 mg/kg PO	2 gm	50-70 mg/kg	50-70 mg/kg	Hepatotoxicity, hyperuricemia
Streptomycin	Vials:	1 gm, 4 gm	20-40 mg/kg IM	15 mg/kg*** IM	1 gm***	25-30 mg/kg IM	25-30 mg/kg	Ototoxicity nephrotoxicity
Ethambutol	Tablets:	100 mg 400 mg	15-25 mg/kg PO	15-25 mg/kg PO	2.5 gm	50 mg/kg	50 mg/kg	Optic neuritis (decreased red-green color discrimination decreased visual acuity), skin rash

* Isoniazid and rifampin are available as a combination capsule containing 150 mg of isoniazid and 300 mg of rifampin.

** A combination of isoniazid, rifampin, and pyrazinamide in a single tablet is being introduced.

*** In persons above age 60 the daily dose of streptomycin should be limited to 10 mg/kg with a maximum dose of 750 mg.

TABLE 6.2 SECOND LINE ANTI–TUBERCULOSIS DRUGS *

Drug	Dosage Forms		Daily Dose In Children and Adults	Maximum Daily Dose In Children and Adults	Major Adverse Reactions	Recommended Regular Monitoring
Capreomycin	Vials:	1 gm	15–30 mg/kg IM	1 gm	Auditory, vestibular and renal toxicity	Vestibular function audiometery, BUN and creatinine
Kanamycin	Vials:	75 mg 500 mg 1 gm	15–30 mg/kg IM	1 gm	Auditory and renal toxicity, rare vestibular toxicity	Vestibular function audiometery, BUN and creatinine
Ethionamide	Tablets:	250 mg	15–20 mg/kg PO	1 gm	Hepatotoxicity, hypersensitivity, GI disturbance	Hepatic enzymes
Para-amino-salicylic acid	Tablets:	500 mg 1 gm	150 mg/kg PO	12 gm	GI disturbance hypersensitivity, hepatotoxicity, sodium load	
Cycloserine	Capsules:	250 mg	15–20 mg/kg PO	1 gm	Psychosis, convulsions, rash	Assessment of mental status

* These drugs are more difficult to use than drugs listed in Table. They should be used only when necessary and should be given and monitored by health providers experienced in their use.

CASE STUDY

A 48-year-old female was picked up after being found unconscious on the sidewalk. Passersby stated the patient drank frequently and lived in the streets. Further history revealed she had recently been complaining of shortness of breath, cough, and blood-tinged sputum. Patient was stabilized and transported. Two weeks after transport the Infection Control Practitioner from the local hospital called to let the ambulance company know that the patient they had transported was just recently diagnosed with tuberculosis. Further review of the EMS run report revealed the paramedics had only worn gloves to care for and transport the patient.

FOLLOW-UP

Q. What other barriers should have been used?

A. Mask, especially when patient displays symptoms suggestive of a respiratory illness. These symptoms in a patient with her social history should alert EMS personnel to the possibility of tuberculosis.

Q. What actions are necessary now?

A.
  a. Hospital has responsibility to notify the ambulance company of potential exposure of their personnel to an infectious disease.
  b. Employer should notify exposed employees.
  c. Employer should provide TB testing now and 6-10 weeks from now.
  d. If employee's skin test converts, he/she should be referred to local health department or agency's Health Care Professional for post-exposure evaluation and follow-up.

Notes

Chapter Seven

Record-keeping

Notes

RECORD KEEPING

A complete infection control program will require several types of recordkeeping.

First, an infection control plan and an exposure control plan (ECP) will need to be written. The development of the ECP requires documentation of the methods and rationale for the contents of the plan as well as the plan itself. Details of these requirements can be found in the Final Rule for Bloodborne Pathogen Standard published December 6, 1991 in the Federal Register and in Chapter 5 of this manual.

The rule requires on-going evaluation (QA) of the effectiveness of the plan, and revisions must be made when new tasks or procedures are identified or any changes in the Rule or information from CDC are published. Records detailing these activities should be maintained.

All exposure incidents are to be investigated and documented and a record of these investigations kept on file.

MEDICAL RECORDS:

OSHA requires that a confidential medical record be maintained for each employee with occupational exposure. This medical record should contain:

- Name and social security number of employee.
- Copy of employee's hepatitis B vaccination status including the dates of all the hepatitis B vaccinations and any medical records relative to the employee's ability to receive [Hep. B] vaccinations.
- Copy of all results of examinations, medical testing, and follow-up procedures [for an exposure incident].
- Employer's copy of the health care professional's written opinion following an exposure incident.

■ Copy of the information provided to the health care professional [following an exposure incident].

The employee's medical record is to be kept confidential and may not be disclosed or reported without the employee's express written consent to anyone within or outside the work place except as required by law.

These records are to be maintained by the employer for at least the duration of employment plus thirty (30) years.

In addition to the above required record keeping, an employer will want to establish a confidential medical record for employees that provides the following voluntary information.

Name and social security number
Emergency information
Person to be notified in event of emergency
Hospital of choice
Personal physician and phone number
Pertinent medical history
Allergies
Medications
Pre-placement physical and health examination
Record of fitness testing for:
1. work,
2. particulate respirators if used
Summary of work related injuries and illnesses
Immunization record
    Measles - verification of immunity or disease
    Mumps - verification of immunity or disease
    Rubella - verification of immunity or disease
    Chicken pox - history of disease
    dT (diphtheria/tetanus) - date of last vaccine
    polio - verification of vaccines
Employer provided vaccines and antibody status
    Hepatitis B - dates of 1, 2, 3rd vaccine; antibody status
    Measles - date of vaccine and/or titer
    Mumps - date of vaccine and/or titer
    Rubella - date of vaccine and/or titer
    Chicken pox - VZ titer
Employer provided surveillance programs
    TB - routine and post-exposure, test results
    Respirator fitness testing

Post exposure evaluation and follow-up including prophylactic treatments (this is in addition to bloodborne pathogen exposures).

Examples of health and medical records are provided at the end of this chapter.

TRAINING RECORDS

OSHA requires that ECP training records include:

- Dates of training session
- Contents or summary of the training sessions
- Names and qualifications of persons conducting training
- Names and job titles of all persons attending the training session

These records should be maintained for at least three (3) years.

The record keeping requirements for training in the Exposure Control Plan would serve nicely for all training programs in infection control, and the authors recommend they be incorporated in the agency's infection central program, including the CDC's new training curriculum for prevention of transmission of tuberculosis. Examples of training records are provided at the end of this chapter.

FIGURE 7.1   HEALTH RECORD

NAME _____ SS# _____

DEPARTMENT _____ POSITION _____

DATE OF PHYSICAL _____ D.O.B. _____

HEPATITIS B SURFACE ANTIBODY: ☐ POSITIVE   ☐ NEGATIVE

Date	X-Rays	Blood Pressure	Weight	CBC	Complete UA	V.Z. Titer	Anti HBS	HBSAG	SGPT	Mumps Titer	Rubeola Riter	Rubella Titer	Mumps Vaccine	Rebeo/Rubella 0.5cc Sub Q	MMR 0.5cc Sub Q	Rubella Vac. 0.5cc Sub Q	Rubeola 0.5cc Sub Q	D.T. Booster 0.5cc IM	Flu Vaccine 0.5cc IM	Mantoux 5PPD 0.1cc Intradermal	Other	HEPATITIS B VACCINE 1CC IM BRAND
																						1st Dose: Date / Site / Sig
																						2nd Dose: Date / Site / Sig
																						3rd Dose: Date / Site / Sig
																						4th Dose: Date / Site / Sig
																						5th Dose: Date / Site / Sig

Recordkeeping

EMPLOYEE REPORT OF INJURY (MUST BE COMPLETED BEFORE END OF SHIFT)

Report below all injuries which arise out of and in the course of employment.

❶ INJURED EMPLOYEE

Name	Dept.			Job Title
Street Address	Sex	Age	Date of Birth	Social Security Number
City		State	Zip	

❷ INJURY OR DISEASE

Incident Date	Date of Report	Time	AM PM

Location of Incident

Description of injury or exposure to occupational hazard; include all pertinent facts.

What was employee doing when injured? How and why did injury occur?

Body Part Injured (Specify)	Equipment Involved (Specify)
Signature of Employee	Witness
Signature of Charge Person	Department Manager Notified Yes ❏ No ❏
Signature of Person Preparing Report	Signature of Employee Receiving Copy of Report

❸ MEDICAL EXAM AFTER INCIDENT

Patient Name*	Room Number	Diagnosis
❏ Refused Medical Treatment		Signature of Employee Refusing Medical Treatment
Date of Treatment		Time AM PM

Treatment

Diagnosis	Estimated Lost Time From Work
Medical Treatment by (Print Name)	Signature of Physician

*If applicable

FIGURE 7.2

FIGURE 7.3

**CONFIDENTIAL RECORD
BLOOD/BODY FLUID EXPOSURE WORKSHEET**

Date _____ Time _____ Run # _____

Employee Name _____ Employee No. _____

Date of Exposure _____ Time of Exposure _____

Name of Source Individual _____ Hospital _____

Results of Source Testing: HIV _____ HBV _____ HCV _____ Other _____

Employee Notified of results and counseled regarding confidentiality on _____

SOURCE OF EXPOSURE:
❑ Spit/Saliva   ❑ Sero-sanguinous Fluid
❑ Blood   ❑ Pus
❑ Urine   ❑ Feces
❑ Vomitus   ❑ Other _____

TYPE OF EXPOSURE:
A. ❑ Skin
    ❑ Puncture, Incision
    ❑ Laceration, Abrasion
    ❑ Eczema
    ❑ Hangnail
    ❑ Pierced ears
    ❑ Needle Stick
    ❑ Open sore, scratches or lesions

B. ❑ Mucous Membrane
    ❑ Eye
    ❑ Nose
    ❑ Mouth

C. ❑ Clothing
    ❑ Soaked
    ❑ Drop(s)
    ❑ Diluted
    ❑ Dried
    ❑ If blood soaks through clothing, Mark A and complete appropriately

MARKING:
1. If A is checked and any area under A was marked, send to HCP for post-exposure evaluation.
2. If B is checked and area under B was exposed, send to HCP for post-exposure evaluation.
3. If C is checked along with A and/or B was checked, send to HCP for post-exposure evaluation.
4. If A is checked, but no area under A is checked, no evaluation needed. File report.
5. If C is checked, but A and B are not, no evaluation is needed. Change contaminated clothing and file report.

DURATION OF EXPOSURE _____ MIN/HR (circle total time)

EXTENT OF EXPOSURE: ❑ Drop(s) of Blood/Body Fluid ❑ Large amount of Blood/Body Fluid

PRECAUTIONS TAKEN: ❑ Gloves ❑ Gauntlets ❑ Goggles ❑ Mask ❑ Faceshield ❑ Gown/Suit

CONCLUSION: Marking ❑ 1 ❑ 2 ❑ 3 ❑ 4 ❑ 5

Disposition:
❑ to counseling on _____ (date)   ❑ to change clothing
❑ to testing on _____ (date)   ❑ Report closed and filed on _____ (date)

Supervisor signature _____ Date _____

CHECKLIST FOR HEALTH CARE PROVIDER
PROVIDING FOLLOW-UP MEDICAL EVALUATION FOR EMPLOYEE OF ...
(COMPANY) ... FOR POSSIBLE EXPOSURE TO A BLOODBORNE PATHOGEN

❑ Received a copy of 29CFR part 1910.1030 OSHA Rule.

❑ Description of employee's duties as they related to the exposure incident.

❑ Results of the source individual's test for blood borne pathogens.

❑ Employee's company medical records.

❑ Employee's vaccination record.

Written opinion must contain the following:

1. Whether it is recommended or not that the employee receive Hepatitis B vaccination.

2. Document that the employee has been informed of:

    a. Results of evaluation.

    b. Any medical condition resulting from the exposure which will require further evaluation or treatment.

Any other unrelated medical condition the evaluation reveals should not be included in medical report to employer and should remain confidential.

Report must be received by employer within 15 days of completion.

_____ (M.D./D.O.)
Signature of physician conducting examination

FIGURE 7.4

FIGURE 7.5

CERTIFICATE OF COURSE COMPLETION

_____ has completed a course in Exposure Control Plan on _____.

I _____ have attended a course of instruction and have read and understand Exposure Control Plan. I understand that I may obtain a copy of this plan by requesting one from my supervisor. I understand that I am to immediately report to my supervisor any known or suspected occupational exposure to blood and/or certain body fluids.

_____   _____
Signature   Date Signed

Recordkeeping

FIGURE 7.6

**SAMPLE
REPORT OF EDUCATION PLAN**

Title of Program _____

Instructor: _____ Date: _____ Time: _____

Employee Name (Print)	Initials	Job Title	Post Test Score
1			
2			
3			
4			
5			
6			
7			
8			
9			
10			
11			
12			
13			
14			
15			
16			
17			
18			
19			
20			
21			

Attach instructor resume; copy of outline; and objectives and skill evaluation check sheets to this form; and maintain for three (3) years.

NOTES

CHAPTER EIGHT

QUALITY ASSURANCE SURVEILLANCE & MONITORING

NOTES

QUALITY ASSURANCE

SURVEILLANCE AND MONITORING

Quality assurance is a system used to establish standards, monitor how well those standards are met and correct unwarranted variations from those standards.

Surveillance is a systematic, active and ongoing observation and documentation of those occurances.

Compliance and quality monitoring are essential components of an effective infection control program. The monitoring process should begin as soon as the program is implemented. A Compliance/Quality Monitoring Program is a requirement published under national guidelines.

CDC Guidelines (MMWR June 1989) "Employers should monitor the work place to ensure that required work practices are observed and that protective clothing and equipment are provided and properly used."

CDC Guidelines (1987) specifically address the need for compliance monitoring. "When non-compliance is noted, the employee should receive counseling, education, and/or training. If this is not effective, appropriate disciplinary action should be considered."

OSHA and CDC, in a Joint Advisory Notice (October 19, 1987) recommended "observed routine surveillance of work place compliance with work practices and use of protective clothing/equipment." This document also states that "non-compliance which is noted should be clearly documented and the corrective action listed."

METHODS

Compliance and quality monitoring can be achieved in a variety of ways.

1) Prospective - performed before the event;

2) Concurrent - performed at the time of the event;

3) Retrospective - performed after the event.

Prospective quality monitoring can be divided into four activities: the initial education, continuing education, periodic skills evaluation to test retention, and a preceptorship program during either education or in response to a perceived or real deficiency delineated during concurrent or retrospective monitoring.

Concurrent (on-scene) monitoring occurs at the time patient care is being given. This can be divided into three areas: direct observation (the most effective method), observation of a preceptorship program, or indirect observation from medical staff upon arrival in the emergency department.

Retrospective monitoring occurs after the fact. EMS run forms (charts) can be reviewed and compliance evaluated by preconceived and documented criteria. Vehicle check list can be retrospectively reviewed for quantity and availability of PPE.

Sample QA forms are provided at the end of this chapter.

FOLLOW-UP PROCESS

If non-compliance is attributed to lack of or inadequate policies and/or procedures, additions and/or revisions should be made. SOPs, engineering and work practice controls should be evaluated, documented, and maintained or replaced on a regular schedule to ensure effectiveness.

Compliance and quality monitoring measures day-to-day effectiveness of your infection control program (Exposure Control Plan). The emphasis is on identifying areas for improvement, problem areas which can be potentially harmful to patients and/or employees and implementing solutions to correct or improve these areas. Ongoing surveillance and quality monitoring are essential and must be in place for an effective infection control program.

FIGURE 8.1 INFECTION CONTROL FIELD AUDIT CHECKLIST

DATE:_____ DIVISION:_____

PERSON CONDUCTING AUDIT:_____

1.	Was daily cleaning accomplished and documented?	YES	NO	N/A
2.	The sharps container easily accessible and secured in upright position.	YES	NO	N/A
3.	The waste container lined with red biohazard bag and secured in upright position.	YES	NO	N/A
4.	Any evidence of food or oral liquids present in the patient compartment.	YES	NO	N/A
5.	The door separating the patient compartment and the cab is closed when a patient is treated or transported.	YES	NO	N/A
6.	Non-sterile gloves readily accessible. a. Quantity - 2 boxes (different size)	YES	NO	N/A
7.	Gowns readily accessible. a. Quantity - 3	YES	NO	N/A
8.	Tyvex suits readily accessible. a. Quantity - 2	YES	NO	N/A
9.	Goggles readily accessible. a. Quantity - 3 pair	YES	NO	N/A
10.	Face shields readily accessible. a. Quantity - 3	YES	NO	N/A
	b. Present with airway equipment.	YES	NO	N/A
11.	Masks readily accessible. a. Quantity - 5	YES	NO	N/A
12.	BVM with mask in Jump Bag.	YES	NO	N/A
13.	Gloves worn when starting IVs.	YES	NO	N/A
14.	Face protection and gloves worn when inserting basic airway adjuncts or when inserting advanced airways.	YES	NO	N/A
15.	Cleaning supplies available on unit. a. Type per current policy	YES	NO	N/A
16.	Hands washed after patient contact.	YES	NO	N/A
17.	Employee can define the following:			
	a. Exposure incident	YES	NO	N/A
	b. Bloodborne pathogen	YES	NO	N/A
	c. Regulated waste	YES	NO	N/A
	d. Universal precaution	YES	NO	N/A
18.	Employee can state the policy and/or procedure to be followed when an exposure incident has occurred.	YES	NO	N/A

FIGURE 8.2

QA MONITORING SUMMARY

Month/Year _____

Important Aspect of Care: Infection Control

INDICATOR	THRESHOLD FOR EVALUATION	SAMPLE SIZE	# IN COMPLIANCE	PERCENT COMPLIANCE	COMMENTS
#1	95%				
#2	100%				
#3	100%				
#4	0%				
#5	95%				
#6	100%				
#7	100%				
#8	100%				
#9	100%				
#10	100%				
#11	100%				
#12	100%				
#13	95%				
#14	95%				
#15	100%				
#16	95%				
#17	90%				
#18	100%				

ADDITIONAL COMMENTS: _____

_____

_____

\# Indicators are taken from Field Audit Checklist

SUBMITTED BY: _____ DATE: _____

CHAPTER NINE

Employee Health & Hygiene Policies & Procedures

- **Pre-placement physical fitness assessment**
- **Recommended immunizations**
- **TB screening**
- **Policies**
  - **Medical records**
  - **Physicals**
  - **TB screening**
  - **Hand washing**
  - **Hair**
  - **Uniforms**
  - **Jewelry/insignias**
  - **Employee illnesses**

Notes

PERSONAL HEALTH & HYGIENE POLICIES & PRACTICES

PRE-PLACEMENT PHYSICAL FITNESS ASSESSMENT

Pre-placement physical fitness assessment is a recommended work practice. The prudent employer will want assurances that the employee has been evaluated and determined to be physically fit to perform the job tasks.

With the signing of the Americans With Disabilities Act (ADA) into law, the process by which physical fitness is determined has been changed. Employers may not require pre-employment physicals but may require a fitness exam after a contingent job offer has been made. This exam must be job specific and used only to determine if the prospective employee is able to perform the essential job tasks.

The Act further requires that an employer make reasonable accommodations for individuals who are unable to perform job tasks due to a disability or perceived disability.

THE PRE-PLACEMENT FITNESS EVALUATION SHOULD INCLUDE:

- evaluation of physical fitness to perform essential job tasks
- evaluation of previous medical history as it relates to person's ability to perform essential job tasks
- immunization history for measles, mumps, rubella, chickenpox, diphtheria, tetanus, polio, hepatitis B
- TB testing

IMMUNIZATION RECOMMENDATIONS FOR ADULT HEALTH CARE WORKERS

The following are the recommendations of the Immunization Practices Advisory Committee, DHHS, USPHS, CDC.

CHICKENPOX "Most persons with a clearly positive history of previous varicella are probably immune. Many with negative or unknown histories may be immune, but some may also be susceptible...Serological screening may be used to define susceptibility." No long term vaccine is available for varicella. [1]

MEASLES "...all health personnel born in 1957 or later who may have contact with patients infected with the measles should be immune. Such persons can be considered immune only if they have documentation of having received two doses of live-measles vaccine after their first birthday, a record of physician-diagnosed measles or laboratory evidence of immunity. Measles vaccine is recommended for all persons lacking such documentation. Combined MMR vaccine is the vaccine of choice if recipients are likely to be susceptible to rubella and/or mumps as well as to measles. Adults born before 1957 can be considered immune to measles..." [2]

MUMPS "While most adults are likely to have been infected naturally with mumps, mumps vaccine may be given to adults, especially males who are considered susceptible." [3]

RUBELLA "... all medical, dental, laboratory and other support health personnel, both male and female, who might be at risk of exposure to patients infected with rubella, or who might have contact with pregnant patients, should be immune. Rubella vaccine is recommended for all such personnel unless they have either proof of vaccination with rubella vaccine on or after their first birthday or laboratory evidence of immunity. Combined MMR vaccine is the vaccine of choice if recipients are likely to be susceptible to measles and/or mumps as well as to rubella." [4]

HEPATITIS B "Persons at substantial risk of HBV infection who are demonstrated or judged likely to be susceptible should be vaccinated. They include all persons with occupational risks. HBV infection is a major infectious occupational hazard for health-care and public-safety workers. The risk of acquiring HBV infection from occupational exposures is dependent on the frequency of percutaneous and permucousal exposures to blood or blood products. Any health-care or public-safety worker may be at risk for HBV exposure depending on tasks that he or she performs. If those tasks involve contact with blood or blood-contaminated body fluids, such workers should be vaccinated." [5]

TETANUS/DIPHTHERIA "All adults...should complete a series of tetanus and diphtheria toxoids. A primary series for adults is three doses of preparations containing tetanus and diphtheria toxoids, with the first two doses given at least 4 weeks apart and the third dose given 6-12 months after the second. Those who have completed a primary series should receive a booster dose every 10 years. The combined toxoids for adult use, Td, should have been used to enhance protection against both diseases. Persons with unknown or uncertain histories of receiving tetanus or diphtheria toxoids should be considered un-immunized and should receive a full three-dose primary series of Td." [6]

NOTE: Prior to the administration of any vaccine, the recipient and the person administering the vaccine should be completely informed regarding "susceptibility of the recipient, the risk of exposure to the disease, the risk from the disease, and the benefits and risk from the immunization agent." [7] An informed consent form should be signed by the recipient prior to receiving immunization. Special precautions and contraindications should be observed with any immuno-suppressed individuals or those who are or may become pregnant during the inoculation process. Individuals refusing to accept vaccinations should be required to sign a refused waiver form.

TB SCREENING

- At the time of employment, all health-care facility personnel, including those with a history of Bacillus of Calmette and Guerin (BCG) vaccination, should receive a Mantoux tuberculin skin test unless a previously positive reaction can be documented or completion of adequate preventive therapy or adequate therapy for active disease can be documented.

- Initial and follow-up tuberculin skin tests should be administered and interpreted according to current guidelines.

- Health-care facility personnel with a documented history of a positive tuberculin test, or inadequate treatment for disease or preventive therapy for infection, should be exempt from further screening unless they develop symptoms suggestive of tuberculosis.

- Periodic re-testing of PPD-negative health-care workers should be conducted to identify persons whose skin tests convert to positive. In general, the frequency of repeat testing should be based on the risk of developing new infection. Health-care facility workers who may be frequently exposed to patients with tuberculosis or who are involved with potentially high-risk procedures (e.g. bronchoscopy, sputum induction, or aerosol treatments given to patients who may have tuberculosis) should be re-tested at least every 6 months. Health-care facility personnel in other areas should be re-tested annually. Data on skin test conversions should be periodically reviewed so that the risk of acquiring new infection may be estimated for each area of the facility. On the basis of this analysis, the frequency of re-testing may be altered accordingly.

Evaluation of health-care-facility personnel after unprotected exposure to tuberculosis

■ In addition to periodic screening, health-care-facility personnel and patients should be evaluated if they have been exposed to a potentially infectious tuberculosis patient for whom the infection-control procedures outlined in this document have not been taken. Unless a negative skin test has been documented within the preceding 3 months, each exposed health-care-facility worker (except those already known to be positive reactors) should receive a Mantoux tuberculin skin test soon as possible after exposure and should be managed in the same way as other contacts. If the initial skin test is negative, the test should be repeated 10-12 weeks after the exposure ended. Exposed persons with skin-test reactions > 5 mm or with symptoms suggestive of tuberculosis should receive chest radiographs. Persons with previously known positive skin-test reactions who have been exposed to an infectious patient do not require a repeat skin test or a chest radiograph unless they have symptoms suggestive of tuberculosis.

Evaluation and management of health-care facility personnel with positive skin tests or symptoms that may be due to tuberculosis

■ Health-care-facility personnel with positive tuberculin skin tests or with skin-test conversions on repeat testing or after exposure should be clinically evaluated for active tuberculosis. Persons with symptoms suggestive of tuberculosis should be evaluated regardless of skin-test results. If tuberculosis is diagnosed, appropriate therapy should be instituted according to published guidelines. Personnel diagnosed with active tuberculosis should be offered counseling and HIV-antibody testing.

■ Health-care-facility personnel who have positive tuberculin skin tests or skin-test conversions but do not have clinical tuberculosis should be evaluated for preventive therapy according to published guidelines. Personnel with positive skin tests should be evaluated for risk of HIV infection. If HIV infection is considered a possibility, counseling and HIV-antibody testing should be strongly encouraged.

■ All persons with a history of tuberculosis or positive tuberculin tests are at risk for contracting tuberculosis in the future. These persons should be reminded periodically that they should promptly report any pulmonary symptoms. If symptoms of tuberculosis should develop, the person should be evaluated immediately.

Routine and follow-up chest radiographs

■ Routine chest films are not required for asymptomatic, tuberculin-negative health-care-facility personnel. After the initial chest radiograph is taken, personnel with positive skin-test reactions do not need repeat chest radiographs unless symptoms develop that may be due to tuberculosis.

Work restrictions

Health-care-facility personnel with current pulmonary or laryngeal tuberculosis pose a risk to patients and other personnel while they are infectious; therefore, stringent work restrictions for these persons are necessary. They should be excluded from work until adequate treatment is instituted, cough is resolved, and sputum is free of bacilli on three consecutive smears. Health-care-facility personnel with current tuberculosis at sites other than the lung or larynx usually do not need to be excluded from work if concurrent pulmonary tuberculosis has been ruled out. Personnel who discontinue treatment before the recommended course of therapy has been completed should not be allowed to work until treatment is resumed, an adequate response to therapy is documented, and they have negative sputum spears on three consecutive days.

- Health-care-facility personnel who are otherwise healthy and receiving preventive treatment for tuberculous infection should be allowed to continue usual work activities.

- Health-care-facility personnel who cannot take or do not accept or complete a full course of preventive therapy should have their work situations evaluated to determine whether reassignment is indicated. Work restrictions may not be necessary for otherwise healthy persons who do not accept or complete preventive therapy. These persons should be counseled about the risk of contracting disease and should be instructed to seek evaluation promptly if symptoms develop that may be due to tuberculosis, especially if they have contact with high-risk patients (i.e. patients at high risk for severe consequences if they become infected).

Consultation

Consultation on tuberculosis surveillance, screening, and other methods to reduce tuberculosis transmission should be available from state health department tuberculosis-control programs. Facilities are encouraged to use the services of health departments in planning and implementing their surveillance and screening programs." [8]

PERSONNEL PRACTICES POLICY STATEMENTS

1. Employee health records will be maintained on all employees while working full or part-time with the company/agency. This record shall include:

    ❑ Pre-placement physical examination

    ❑ Immunization record

    ❑ Surveillance/screening results

- ❏ Record of employee exposures to infectious diseases and course of treatment per OSHA

- ❏ Special health considerations or incidents

- ❏ Work related injuries and course

- ❏ Other _____
    Specify

2. A pre-placement physical fitness assessment will be completed prior to assignment to job tasks.

3. Routine yearly TB skin testing will be required for all employees having contact with patients. For those individuals who have converted their skin tests, this policy will be waived. Instead, an initial chest x-ray will be obtained and appropriate counseling provided regarding the need to report any signs or symptoms of TB. Further chest x-rays will only be obtained when determined necessary by the consulting physician.

4. Frequent hand washing is required. Hands will be washed when you arrive at work, before and after each patient contact, after using the restroom facility, before and after eating, after smoking, after use of a handkerchief or tissue, after touching any body hair, and before and after any invasive procedure, after removal of PPE and before entering the cab of the vehicle.
    Hand washing is the single most important means of preventing the spread of infection in the prehospital care setting. Therefore, it is important to know where and how to wash your hands. When a hand washing facility is not available, employees are to use an approved hand cleanser provided in the vehicle.

POLICY STATEMENT:

1. Hands shall be washed when you arrive at work.
2. Hand shall be washed before and after each patient contact, after removing PPE and before entering cab of vehicle.
3. Hands shall be washed after you go to the restroom, before and after eating, after smoking, or use of handkerchief or tissue, and before and after any invasive procedure.

PROCEDURE FOR WASHING THE HANDS WHEN HAND WASHING FACILITIES ARE AVAILABLE

1. Wet your hands under running water.
2. Keeping hands lower than elbows apply soap to hands.
3. Scrub into lather using rotation, frictional motion, scrubbing fingers, backs of hands, wrists, forearms and under the nails for at least 15 second after lather.

Employee Health & Hygiene Policies & Procedures

4. Thoroughly rinse hands under running water making sure the water runs from your fingers to your elbows.
5. Use paper towels to blot and dry the hands.
6. Use paper towels to turn off the faucets and discard towels in receptacle.

PROCEDURE FOR WASHING THE HANDS WHEN HAND WASHING FACILITIES ARE NOT AVAILABLE

1. Apply designated cleanser to hands, thoroughly saturating fingers, hands and wrists. Allow 15 seconds contact time.
2. Follow manufacturer's recommendations for any product of this nature.
3. Under no circumstances should an individual exceed six (6) applications without undertaking a thorough hand washing procedure using an appropriate hand washing facility.

HAIR

Hair must at all times be neat and secured away from the face. Long hair must be secured and not permitted to fall forward or onto the shoulders. Facial hair, specifically beards, should not be permitted due to the fact they have been demonstrated to enhance bacterial growth and contamination. While some authors would suggest that beards may be permitted, provided full face hoods are available for the personnel to wear when needed, the efficacy of this for pre-hospital care providers makes this an impractical approach. Further, studies have suggested that the full face/head hoods may actually contribute to an increase in microbial growth and spread when removed. [9]

FOR THIS REASON, WE RECOMMEND THAT:

1. No beards be permitted.
2. If mustaches are permitted, they must be trimmed and not be permitted to extend below the upper lip or corner of the mouth.
3. Sideburns should be short and not permitted to extend past the earlobe.
4. If particulate respirators are used, personel required to wear respirators will not be permitted beards or mustaches, as this hair will interfere with an effective seal of the mask on the face.

Personnel must avoid touching their hair. If the hair is touched with the hands, the hands must be washed prior to patient contact.

POLICY STATEMENT

Hair shall be clean and neatly secured away from the face and not permitted to fall forward on the neck or shoulders. Hair must be maintained so as to prevent contamination of a patient's open skin or mucous membranes or any susceptible patient. Employees must refrain from touching their hair while engaging in patient care and if the hair is touched, hands must be washed prior to patient contact. Beards are not permitted. Mustaches will be permitted provided they are kept clean and neatly trimmed and not permitted to extend below the level of the upper lip, or to interfere in obtaining a seal when wearing a particulate respirator. Sideburns will be permitted provided they are kept clean and neatly trimmed and are not permitted to extend below the level of the earlobe. If particular respirators are used, personnel required to wear particular respirators should not be permitted mustaches.

UNIFORMS

Each agency will want to designate for itself the type and style of uniform its employees will wear. It is recommended that when selecting uniforms, the company will consider washability and stain resistance in addition to appearance. All parts of the uniform including outerwear must be able to be cleaned on a regular basis.

In addition to the standard uniform, the company/agency will need to identify the type of protective garments to be worn by their personnel when conditions indicate their use. This will include, but not be limited to, masks, full length gowns with long sleeves or jumpsuits, or fluid resistant coats and pants, gloves, eye protection (goggles, glasses with side and top shields or face shields) and possible booties and hair coverings when necessary.

Our experience has shown that disposable garments are the most advantageous at this time. If non-disposable garments are selected, a special procedure will need to be developed that describes who will handle these garments and how they will be laundered.

Agencies will need to develop a policy regarding clean uniforms. This policy should state that a clean uniform will be worn each working shift and that should the uniform become soiled with patient's blood or body fluids, the uniform will immediately be changed. These policies will help ensure that the uniform does not become a source of contamination or infection both for your patients and your employees. The soiled uniform is not to be taken home, but must be washed either using an in-agency laundry facility or outside laundry/dry cleaning facility.

POLICY STATEMENT

Designated uniforms will be worn by all personnel having contact with patients. This uniform is to be worn only while on duty. PPE including outerwear protection is to be worn anytime there is an opportunity for blood and/or body fluids to splash, spray or come in contact with uniform.

See Isolation Techniques for specific information regarding Universal Precautions and the use of barrier techniques.

Uniforms that become soiled with a patient's excretions, secretions, blood and/or body fluids will be changed immediately and placed in biohazard linen container. An incident report will be completed by the employee, describing the circumstances surrounding the incident that caused the uniform to become contaminated. A supervisor will complete a follow-up investigation and make recommendations on how to prevent a recurrence.

JEWELRY/INSIGNIA

In general, jewelry should not be permitted to be worn while on duty with the exception of approved uniform insignia and medic alert tags. Necklaces that are worn under the clothing may also be permitted. Watches are permitted as a part of the approved uniform, however, they must be kept clean, and there will be times when you will wish to remove the watch rather than permit it to become contaminated. Contaminated jewelry will need to be disinfected as with any other type of non-disposable equipment. Rings are a serious source of contamination. They cause moisture and debris to become trapped beneath them, thus permitting growth of microbes. For this reason rings should not be permitted to be worn while on duty nor while caring for patients.

POLICY STATEMENT

Only approved jewelry/insignia will be permitted to be worn while on duty and involved in delivery of patient care. Approved jewelry/insignia can be found in the company policy and procedure manual under uniform section. If not addressed in that section, watches will be permitted to be worn while on duty, however, it is the responsibility of the employee to prevent contamination of the watch, and in the event the watch becomes contaminated, it is the responsibility of the employee to disinfect/clean this item.

EMPLOYEE ILLNESSES

It should be obvious to all providers that employees who attempt to work when they are ill pose a hazard to both other employees and to the patients we are charged with caring for, and in many situations create more problems by being at work than if they had chosen to call in sick. Therefore, in general employees who are sick should not be permitted to work. There are exceptions to this rule and for the most part these are described in the chapter titled Employee Exposures and Illnesses.

As a guideline, employees with elevated temperatures, sore throats, symptoms of respiratory infections, any draining lesions or diarrhea should be referred to their supervisor before being permitted to have patient contact. Employees who have active infections are to have no contact with patients or shall use adequate protective devices and procedures while on duty.

Employees who have been off work three (3) or more days with an illness should be required to submit a return to work note signed by a physician prior to returning to work.

POLICY STATEMENT

Employees who have active infections are to have no patient contact until evaluated by a physician and determined to be able to resume job duties. Employees with specific infectious conditions will be required to wear protective devices and be prohibited from specific procedures as deemed appropriate by consulting physician and expert panel. These devices/procedures are described in the chapter titled Employee Exposures and Illnesses. No employee with weeping or draining lesions on the hands will be permitted to engage in patient care. In addition, the supervisor will ensure that a Workman's Compensation record is initiated by the employee if applicable.

Chapter Ten

Disaster Implications

NOTES

Natural Disasters and Infection Control

Control of patients, contacts and the immediate environment is important in given situations where diseases might constitute a problem in a disaster situation. There may be the need for preventive measures. The following diseases may have disaster implications.

ACQUIRED IMMUNODEFICIENCY SYNDROME
All health care providers should follow universal precautions when providing care to patients of disasters. If blood transfusions are needed, blood that has been pre-screened for HIV antibodies should be used.

AMEBIASIS
An outbreak of Amebiasis may occur if there is a disruption of sanitary facilities.

ANTHRAX
In flood disasters where there were previously infected areas.

CAMPYLOBACTERIOSIS (Diarrhea caused by camphlobacter)
May be a risk if there is poor sanitation existing when food is being delivered to a large group of people.

CHICKENPOX - Herpes Zoster
Outbreak risk in areas where it is endemic and if there are large groups of people. Sanitary facilities and safe food handling are recommended.

COCCIDIOIDOMYCOSIS
In dusty conditions where groups of susceptible people are traveling through may be a possible hazard.

DENGUE FEVER
In situations of hurricanes or severe tropical storms, large, extensive epidemics can occur.

DIPHTHERIA
In conditions where crowding (especially infants and children), outbreaks can be a problem.

VIRAL HEPATITIS A
There may be a problem in large groups of people where there is poor sanitation and inadequate water supplies. May need to improve sanitation and ensure safe water supplies. Administration of IG in mass is not recommended as a substitute for ensuring safe environmental measures.

VIRAL HEPATITIS B
Universal precautions should be followed by health care providers when treating patients in disaster situations. If possible screen blood prior to transfusions to minimize the number of cases.

VIRAL HEPATITIS C
Same as Hepatitis B

DELTA HEPATITIS
Same as Hepatitis B

HEPATITIS E
Same as Hepatitis A

HISTOPLASMOSIS
Potential for acute pulmonary diseases may occur in an endemic area. May be complicated if there is a history of dust in a closed space. Also suspect places such as barns, chicken coops, silos, blackbird roosts, starling roosts and attics or basements.

INFLUENZA
If the virus is introduced in shelters where emergency housing has large numbers of people, there is the likelihood for an outbreak.

LEPROSY
Interruption of scheduled treatments may be a serious problem.

LEPTOSPIROSIS
In areas where there is a high water table and flooding occurs there may be a potential problem.

MALARIA
Breeding sites in endemic areas where the climate may change may increase the mosquito populations and an increase in malaria.

MEASLES
Devastating epidemics can occur when there is an introduction of measles to susceptible people in refugees/camps.

MENINGITIS
In situations where a large group of people are required to be housed together, epidemics may develop.

PERTUSSIS
In refugee camps non-immunized children may have a problem with pertussis.

PLAGUE
In situations of social upheavals where there are large groups of people living in poor hygienic conditions, Plague could become a problem.

PNEUMONIA
The elderly are especially at risk in situations where there are large numbers of people living in temporary shelters.

POLIOMYLITIS
An epidemic threat may occur where there are non-immune, overcrowded groups of people.

RABIES
In areas where there are stray dogs or wild animals, there is a potential problem of this disease.

RELAPSING FEVER
Epidemics are common in situations such as wars or where overcrowding of malnourished populations exist with poor hygiene. To prevent this disease, suggest to those traveling into tick infested areas that they wear clothes that cover as much skin as possible. Sleeves and collars should be snug fitting and pants tucked into boots.

SALMONELLOSIS
In situations with poor sanitation and mass feeding occurs, there may be a danger.

SCABIES
In overcrowded areas Scabies may be a potential nuisance.

SHIGELLOSIS
In situations where personal hygiene is poor and the environment is poor, there may be a potential problem.

SMALLPOX
A major disaster may occur if the virus is introduced into a non-immune populated area unless quickly controlled.

STREPTOCOCCAL DISEASE
Patients with wounds such as thermal burns are highly susceptible to an infection at the wound site.

TETANUS
Traumatic injuries in disaster situations where there are non-immune populations may result in an increased need for TIG or tetanus antitoxins and toxoid for victims.

TRENCH FEVER
In crowded shelters with poor hygiene, there is an increased risk.

TYPHOID FEVER
Transmission may occur if there are active cases in populations where there is a disruption in the water supply or sewage disposal.

EPIDEMIC LOUSEBORNE TYPHUS FEVER
In louse-infested populations where a large group of people are living, Typhus can be a significant problem.

MURINE TYPHUS FEVER
When humans are forced to live among rats and fleas there may be a problem.

ABBREVIATIONS

AIDS Acquired Immune Deficiency Syndrome.

BBP Bloodborne Pathogens

CDC Centers for Disease Control

DOL Department of Labor

HBV Hepatitis B Virus

HCV Hepatitis C Virus

HHS Department of Health and Human Services

HIV Human Immune Deficiency Virus, causative agent for AIDS

IM Intramuscular

MMR Measles, mumps, rubella vaccine

MMWR Morbidity and Mortality Weekly Report – a publication of CDC

OPIM Other potentially infectious material

OSHA Occupational Safety and Health Act/Administration

PPE Personal Protective Equipment

SQ Subcutaneous

TB Tuberculosis

Glossary of Terms

Acute (disease)	of short duration, usually with an abrupt onset and sometimes severe (as opposed to chronic disease).
AIDS (Acquired Immunodeficiency Syndrome)	the most severe manifestation of infection with the human immunodeficiency virus (HIV).
Airborne	a means of spreading pathogenic microorganisms from the respiratory tract which may be discharged from the nose or mouth by coughing, sneezing or talking.
Amniotic fluid	the watery fluid that surrounds the fetus or unborn child in the uterus.
Antibiotic	any of a variety of substances both natural and synthetic which inhibit the growth of or destroy microorganisms.
Antibody	substance that a person's immune system develops to help fight infection.
Antibody positive	the result of a test or series of tests to detect antibodies in blood. A positive result means that antibodies are present.
Antigen	substance such as HIV that is foreign to a person's body. An antigen causes the immune system to form antibodies to fight the antigen.
Antitoxin	an antibody capable of neutralizing a specific toxin.
Antiviral drug	a drug that can interfere with the life cycle of a virus.
ARC (AIDS-Related Complex or Condition)	a term that has been used to describe a variety of symptoms caused by HIV infection. These symptoms are usually less severe than those associated with AIDS and can include loss of appetite, weight loss, fever, night sweats, skin rashes, diarrhea, tiredness, lack of resistance to infection, and swollen lymph nodes.
Asymptomatic seropositive	having a disease-causing agent in the body but showing no outward signs of disease.

Asymptomatic HIV	the condition of testing positive for HIV antibody without showing any symptoms of disease. A person who is HIV-positive even without symptoms is capable of transmitting the virus to others.
AZT	the first FDA-approved drug used to treat AIDS.
Bacteria	Unicellular plantlike microorganisms lacking chlorophyll.
Body fluids	fluids that the body makes, for example semen, blood, vaginal secretions, and breast milk.
Blood and body fluid precautions	a means of preventing the spread of disease causing agents which are spread by any body fluid including blood, urine, tears, semen, CSF, etc.
Carrier	a person who apparently is healthy, but who is infected with some disease causing organism (such as HIV or HBV) that can be transmitted to another person.
Centers for Disease Control (CDC)	federal health agency that is a branch of the U.S. Department of Health and Human Services. The CDC provides national health and safety guidelines and statistical data on AIDS and other diseases.
Chronic (disease)	lasting a long time, or recurring often.
Clean	free of any obvious debris.
Culture	a mass of microorganisms growing in laboratory culture media.
Cytomegalovirus (CMV)	a viral infection that may occur without any symptoms or result in mild flu-life symptoms. Severe CMV infections can result in hepatitis, mononucleosis or pneumonia. CMV is "shed" in body fluids (urine, semen, sputum and saliva). In the presence of immune deficiency, such as AIDS, it can also affect other internal organs and vision, sometimes leading to blindness.
Decontamination	removing disease-causing agents, thus making the environment or specific object safe to handle.
Diagnosis	identifying a disease by its signs, symptoms, course and laboratory findings.

Glossary of Terms

Direct contact	a means of spreading disease by direct transmission of bacteria from one person to another.
Disease	a pathological condition of the body that presents a group of symptoms peculiar to it and which sets the condition apart as an abnormal entity differing from other normal or pathological body states.
Drainage/secretion precautions	a means of preventing the spread of disease causing agents which are spread by the sputum, pus, etc.
Droplet contact	infectious agents that may come in contact with the conjunctiva, nose or mouth of a susceptible individual as a result of coughing, sneezing or talking by an infected person.
Elisa test	a screening test for the presence of antibodies to HIV. A positive result from an Elisa test always needs to be confirmed by a second Elisa test and a more specific test.
Enteric precautions	a means of preventing the spread of disease causing agents which are spread by the food-borne route.
Epidemiology	the study of the incidence, distribution and control of a disease in a population.
Etiology	the causes or origins of disease.
Exposure	the act or condition of coming in contact with, but not necessarily being infected by, a disease-causing agent.
False negative	incorrect test result indicating that no antibodies are present when they are.
False positive	incorrect test result indicating that antibodies are present when they are not.
HBIG	hepatitis B immune globulin which is a preparation that provides some temporary protection following exposure to HBV if given within 7 days after exposure.
Helper/suppressor T-cells	white blood cells that are part of the immune system.
Hepatitis B	a viral infection that affects the liver. The effects of the disease on the liver can range from mild, even non-apparent, to severe or fatal.

High-risk behavior	a term that describes certain activities that increase the risk of transmitting HIV or HBV. These include anal intercourse, vaginal intercourse without a condom, oral-anal contact, semen in the mouth, sharing intravenous needles, intimate blood contact.
HIV antibody screening test	a blood test that reveals the presence of antibodies to HIV.
HIV	(human immunodeficiency virus) the cause of AIDS.
HIV antibody positive	a test result indicating that HIV antibodies are found.
HIV antigen positive	the result of antigen testing where it has been found that HIV is present. Antigen testing can be useful in predicting the progression of HIV infection and monitoring treatment.
HIV disease	the term to describe the spectrum of HIV infection, chronologically described as a progression from asymptomatic seropositive to AIDS.
Immune	protected or exempt from disease.
Immune status	the state of the body's immune system. Factors affecting immune status include heredity, age, diet, and physical and mental health.
Immune system	a body system that helps resist disease-causing germs, viruses, or other infections.
Immunizations	a means by which an individual becomes immune or the process of rendering a patient immune.
Immunosuppressed	a condition or state in which the immune system does not work normally.
Incubation period	the time period between infection and appearance of disease symptoms.
Indirect contact	a means of spreading diseases through the use of an intermediary person, thing, animal, flea or tick.
Infection	a condition or state of the body in which a disease-causing agent has entered it.
Intravenous drugs	drugs injected by needle directly into a vein.

Glossary of Terms

ISG	gamma globulin obtained from pooled blood donors' plasma obtained from many donors.
Latency	a period when a virus is in the body but is inactive
Microorganism	minute living body not perceptible to the naked eye.
MMWR	(Morbidity and Mortality Weekly Report) a CDC weekly publication that gives information on current trends in the nation's health.
Mucous membrane	a moist layer of tissue that lines the mouth, eyes, nostrils, vagina, anus, or urethra.
Nonintact skin	skin that is chapped, abraded, weeping, or that has rashes or eruptions.
Opportunistic infection	infection that usually is warded off by a healthy immune system. If the immune system is not strong and effective, these infections take the opportunity to harm the body.
Parenteral	means of transmission (such as needlestick) through the vehicle of blood.
Pathogen	a disease-causing substance
Pathogenic	capable of causing disease.
Percutaneously	entering the body through the skin, for example, by needlestick or on broken skin.
Pericardial fluid	a clear fluid contained in the thin, membranous sac that surrounds the heart.
Perinatal	happening just before, during, or immediately after birth.
Peritoneal fluid	fluid contained in the membrane lining of the abdominal cavity.
Person with AIDS (PWA)	a preferred term for a person diagnosed with AIDS.
Pleural fluid	fluid contained in the membrane that covers the lung and lines the chest cavity.
Pneumocystis carinii Pneumonia (pcp)	a lung infection that has been common among people infected with HIV or diagnosed with AIDS.

Prophylactic	agents which are used to ward off disease.
Prophylaxis	any substance or steps taken to prevent something from happening (for example, condoms, vaccines)
Respiratory isolation	a means of preventing the spread of disease causing agents which are contacted by the airborne route.
Safe sex	sexual practices that involve no exchange of blood, semen, or vaginal secretions.
Seroconversion	the process by which a person previously known to be antibody negative converts to testing positive for HIV antibodies.
Serologic test	any number of tests that are performed on blood. Usually refers to a test that measures antibodies to a virus.
Seropositive	a condition in which antibodies to a disease-causing agent are found in the blood: a positive reaction to a blood test. The presence of antibodies indicates that a person has been exposed to the agent.
Sputum	a substance that is expelled by coughing or clearing the throat and could contain such things as mucus, pus, blood and microorganisms.
Sterilization	destruction of all microbial life by means of steam, gas, or liquid agents.
Strict isolation	a means of preventing the spread of disease-causing agents which could be airborne as well as capable of spreading disease by inanimate objects or surfaces.
Subcutaneous	beneath or introduced beneath the skin (for example, subcutaneous injections).
Syndrome	a collection of signs and symptoms that occur together.
Terminal cleaning	cleaning all receptacles, equipment, floors, furniture, walls and/or airing, disposing of disposable items after each patient use.
Titer	a specific test used as a standard of strength to determine whether a specific amount of antibodies are present in an antiserum.

Toxin	a poisonous substance of animal or plant origin.
Tuberculocidal	capable of killing a moderately resistant bacterium. Mycobacterium tuberculosis var. bovis. This organism is one used in laboratory tests to classify disinfectant chemicals according to their power.
Vaccine	a substance that produces or increases immunity and protection against a particular disease.
Vectorborne	an arthropod (insect or tick) which transmits the causative organisms of disease from infected to noninfected individuals.
Vehicles	an inanimate object (usually blood, water, milk, or biological products) which transmits the causative organisms of disease from infected to non-infected persons or animals.
Virus	organism that causes disease.
Western blot test	a blood test used to detect antibodies to HIV. The test can be used to confirm Elisa test results (see Elisa test).
Window period	the time it takes the immune system to develop antibodies to the virus after exposure to it.

NOTES

BIBLIOGRAPHY

A Curriculum Guide For Public Safety and Emergency Response Workers: Prevention of Transmission of Human Immunodeficiency Virus and Hepatitis B Virus. U.S. Department of Health and Human Services (NIOSH) Publication No. 89-108.

AMA Policy for Testing HIV. *JAMA* February 12, 1992, Vol 267, No 6. 792.

Benenson, Abram S. (Ed.) *Control Of Communicable Diseases In Man,* (15th ed.). Washington, D.C.: American Public Health Association, 1990.

Centers for Disease Control. Public Health Service Guidelines for Counseling and Antibody Testing to Prevent HIV Infection and AIDS, *MMWR* 1987; vol 36/No 31:509-514.

Centers for Disease Control. Prevention and Control of Tuberculosis in Migrant Farm Workers, Recommendations of the Advisory Council for the Elimination of Tuberculosis. *MMWR* 1992, 41(No.RR-10): 1-15.

Centers for Disease Control. Recommendations for preventing transmission of human immunodeficiency virus and hepatitis B virus to patients during exposure-prone invasive procedures. *MMWR* 1991; 40(No. RR-8):1-9.

Centers for Disease Control. Update: Human Immunodeficiency Virus Infections in Health Care Workers Exposed to Blood of Infected Patients. *MMWR* 1987; Vol. 36/No. 19. 285-288.

Centers for Disease Control. Prevention and control of tuberculosis in U.S. communities with at-risk minority populations: recommendations of the Advisory Council for the Elimination of Tuberculosis and Prevention and control of tuberculosis among homeless persons: recommendations of the Advisory Council for the Elimination of Tuberculosis. *MMWR* 1992;41(RR-5):1-23.

Centers for Disease Control. Prevention and control of tuberculosis in migrant farm workers, recommendations of the advisory council for the elimination of tuberculosis. *MMWR* 1992;41(No. RR-10):1-15.

Centers for Disease Control. Revision of the CDC Surveillance Case Definition for Acquired Immunodeficiency Syndrome. *MMWR* 1987;36(suppl no. 1S):1-155.

Centers for Disease Control. Adult Immunization: Recommendations of the Immunization Practices Advisory Committee. *MMWR* Sept. 18, 1984; Vol. 33(suppl no. 1S):15-68S.

Centers for Disease Control. Guidelines for preventing the transmission of tuberculosis in health-care settings, with special focus on HIV-related issues. *MMWR* 1990;39(no. RR-17):1-29.

Centers for Disease Control. Measles prevention: recommendations of the Immunization Practices Advisory Committee (ACIP). *MMWR* 1989(no. S-9):1-18.

Centers for Disease Control. Protection against viral hepatitis: recommendations of the Immunization Practices Advisory Committee (ACIF) *MMWR* 1990;39(No. RR-2):1-26.

Centers for Disease Control. Recommendations for preventing transmission of human immunodeficiency virus and hepatitis B virus to patients during exposure-prone invasive procedures. *MMWR* 1991;40(No. RR-8):1-9.

Centers for Disease Control. Recommendations for prevention of HIV transmission in health-care settings. *MMWR* 1987;36 (suppl no. 2S):1-185.

Centers for Disease Control. Guidelines for Prevention of Transmission of Human Immunodeficiency Virus and Hepatitis B Virus to Health-Care and Public-Safety Workers. *MMWR* 1989;38(no. S-6):1-37.

Centers for Disease Control. Public Health Service Guidelines for Counseling and Antibody Testing to Prevent HIV Infection and AIDS. *MMWR*, August 14, 1987, Vol 36, No 31. 509-515.

Farizo, MD, Karen M., et al. *JAMA*, April 1, 1992, Vol 267, No. 13: Spectrum of Disease in Persons With Human Immunodeficiency Virus Infection in the United States. 1798-1805.

Friedland, MD, Gerald H. & Klein, MD, Robert S., Transmission of the Human Immunodeficiency Virus. *The New England Journal of Medicine.* October 29, 1987 Vol 317 No 18. 1125-1135.

Garner, RN, MS, Julia S. & Simmons, MD, Bryan P. July 1983. CDC Guideline for Isolation Precautions in Hospitals. *Guidelines for Prevention and Control of Nosocomial Infections.* U.S. Dept of Health and Human Services; Public Health Service; Centers For Disease Control.

Isolation Techniques for use in Hospitals. Government Printing Office, Washington D.C. 20402. Supt. Doc. Stock # 017-023-00094-2. Second Edition 1975. Table 102-103.

Lo, MD, Bernard & Steinbrook, MD, Robert. *JAMA*, Feb. 26, 1992, Vol 267, No. 8. Health Care Workers Infected With the Human Immunodeficiency Virus. 1100-1105.

Quinn, T.C. (1990, March). "The Epidemiology of the Human Immunodeficiency Virus." *Annals of Emergency Medicine.* 19. 225-232.

Rutala, W.A. (1990, April). APIC Guideline for Selection and Use of Disinfectants. *American Journal of Infection Control.* 18(2). 99-113.

Sattar, Syed A. & Springthorpe, V. Susan. *Reviews of Infectious Diseases* 1991;13:430-47: Survival and Disinfectant Inactivation of the Human Immunodeficiency Virus: A Critical Review. 430-445.

Update: Acquired Immunodeficiency Syndrome - United States. *MMWR*, January 17, 1986/Vol 35/No 2. 17-21.

U.S. Department of Labor. OSHA 3130 1992: *Occupational Exposure to Bloodborne Pathogens: Precautions for Emergency Responders.* 1-20.

U.S. Department of Labor. OSHA Instruction CPL 2-2.4C (March 6, 1992). Office of Health Compliance Assistance: Enforcement Procedures for the Occupational Exposure to Bloodborne Pathogens Standard, 29 CFR 1910.1030. 1-71.

Williams, MD, MPH, Walter W. July 1983, CDC Guideline For Infection Control in Hospital Personnel. *CDC Guidelines for Prevention and Control of Nosocomial Infections.* Dept of Health and Human Services; Public Health Service; Centers For Disease Control.

Zimmerman, L., Neuman, M., & Farr, P. (1985) *Infection Control Procedures for Prehospital Care Providers.* Grand Rapids, MI: Mercy Ambulance & Saint Mary's Hospital.

INDEX

AAA - American Ambulance Association **118**
AFB isolation **37**
AIDS **18, 39, 51, 81–84, 112–113, 115–120, 161, 165–166, 225**
Abscess - see wound **41, 51**
Acquired immune deficiency syndrome (AIDS) **18, 39, 51, 81–84, 112–113, 115–120, 161, 164, 165–166, 225**
Actinomycosis **51**
Adenoviruses **51**
Airborne transmission **18, 175–176**
Airways **129**
Algorithm for blood exposures **112–113**
Amebiasis **51, 225**
Amebic dysentery **43**
American Ambulance Association - Position Statement **118**
Amniotic fluid **23**
Anthrax **41, 51, 225**
Anti HBs **84, 112–113**
Aplastic anemia **18**
Arthropod, transmission by **18**
Arthropod-borne viral infections **39, 52**
Ascariasis **52**
Aseptic meningitis **62**
Babesiosis **39, 52, 87–88, 169**
Backboards **129**
Bag/valve/mask **129**
Bandages **120, 130**
Barrier techniques **25–32**
Bedpans **129**
Bench, squad **130**
Biohazard **21, 125, 146**
Bite blocks **129**
Blastomycosis **52**

Blood and body fluids **23, 33, 39–40, 47, 112–113**
Blood pressure cuffs (B/P cuffs) **130**
Bloodborne disease(s) **23, 81–96, 115, 159–174**
Bloodborne pathogen(s) **23, 81–96, 115, 159–174**
Booties **31–32**
Botulism **52, 58**
Bronchiolitis **52**
Bronchitis **35, 52**
Brucellosis **39, 41, 53, 88–89, 169**
Bubonic plague **18, 42, 105**
Bulb syringe **130**
Burn infection **36, 41, 53**
CDC **13, 23, 115, 120**
CMV **42, 56, 82, 101**
CardiO2 **131**
Campylobacter **43, 53, 58, 92, 96, 225**
Cancer **18**
Candida albicans – see candidiasis
Candidiasis **53, 81**
Carrier **17, 108**
Case study **121–122, 153–154, 191–192**
Cat scratch fever **53**
Category specific isolation **33–44**
Catheters **131**
Cellulitis **41, 53**
Centers for Disease Control and Prevention (CDC) **13, 23, 115, 120**
Cervical collars **130**
Chancroid **53**
Chickenpox **17, 53, 92, 96–97, 214, 225**
Childhood diseases (illnesses) **96–99**
Chlamydia **53, 65**
Cholera **43, 53**
Cleaning **123–136, 143**
Closed cavity infection **42, 53**
Clostridium **42, 43, 53, 58**
Clothing **128**
Coccidiodomycosis **53, 225**

Index

Cold(s) **35, 54, 99–100**
Cold Packs **130**
Cold sore **47**
Colorado tick fever **18, 39, 53, 89–90, 170**
Combi-tubes **130**
Communication of hazards **146–148, 159–174**
    Labels and signs **146**
    Training **147–148, 159–174**
Conjunctivitis **35, 41, 55, 100**
Contact transmission **17, 33**
Contaminated
    items **125**
    articles **21**
    disposable items **21**
    equipment **21**
    instruments **21**
Coronavirus **55**
Corticosteroids **18**
Counseling **84, 85, 87, 102, 103, 112–113, 116, 117**
Coxsackievirus disease **43, 55**
Creutzfeldt-Jakob disease **39, 55, 61, 90, 171**
Crichothyrotomy kits **130**
Crimean-Congo fever **35, 91–92, 172**
Croup **35, 55**
Cryptococcus **55, 81**
Cryptosporidium **43, 58, 81**
Cysticercosis **55**
Cytomegalovirus (CMV) **42, 56, 82, 101**
Decubitus ulcer **41, 56**
Delta Hepatitis **60, 86, 167, 226**
Dengue **56, 226**
Diarrhea **43, 47, 56**
Dientamoeba fragilis **43, 58**
Diphtheria **35, 56, 101, 214, 226**
Disaster implications **223–228**
Disease specific isolation **49–74**
Disinfection **123–136**

    High level **127**
    Intermediate level **127**
    Low level **128**
    Environmental level **128**
Drainage and secretion precautions **33, 41–42**
Draining wounds **47**
Dressings **130**
Droplet contact **17**
Droplet nuclei **18, 37, 110, 174, 175, 176**
Drug box **130**
EMS **23**
EOA **131**
EPA **127**
Ebola fever (virus) **35, 91–92, 172**
Echinococcosis **56**
Echovirus **43, 56**
Eczema vaccinia **56**
Electrical equipment **132**
Emesis basin **130**
Employee health **79, 211–222**
    Employee illnesses **79–114, 115–120, 221–222**
    Employee exposures **79–114**
    Employee with chronic or life-threatening illness **115–120**
Encephalitis **43, 56**
Endometritis **35, 42, 57, 69**
End tidal carbon dioxide monitor **130, 132**
Endotracheal tube **130**
Engineering controls **141–142**
Enteric precautions **33, 43–44**
Enterobiasis **57**
Enterocolitis **43, 57**
Enteroviral **43, 57**
Environmental Protection Agency – See EPA
Epidemiology **175**
Epiglottitis **37, 57**
Epstein-Barr virus **57**
Erysipeloid **57**

Index

Erythema infectiosum **37, 57**
Escherichia coli (E Coli) **43, 57, 58**
Expert Panel **116**
Exposure control plan **21, 137–152, 185–186**
Exposure incident **145–146**
External cardiac compressor **131**
Eye protection **27–28**
Eye wear **27–28**
Faceshield **26, 27–28**
Fever **47, 57**
Fifth disease **37**
Food poisoning **58**
Furunculosis **35, 42, 58**
Gangrene **42, 58**
Gastroenteritis **43, 59, 101–102**
Gastrointestinal illnesses **43, 44, 58, 59, 101–102**
German measles – See rubella
Giardia lamblia **44, 58, 59, 102**
Gloves **21, 23, 25, 26, 35, 37, 39, 41, 43**
Goggles **21, 24, 27**
Gonococcal opthalmia neonatorum **59**
Gonorrhea **59**
Gown **21, 24, 28–29**
Granulocytopenia **59**
Granuloma inguinale **59**
Guillian-Barre Syndrome **59**
HBIG **112–113**
HBsAg **84–85, 112–113, 163**
HBV – See hepatitis type B
HCV – See hepatitis type C
HCW **115–120**
HIV **18, 61, 81–84, 112–113, 115–120, 139**
HTLV-1 **92, 172**
Haemophilus influenzae (H flu) **65, 105**
Hair **219–220**
Hand, foot and mouth disease **44, 59**
Handwashing **21, 141, 218–219**

Head protection **31–32**
Health care professional **23, 115–120**
Hemorrhagic fever, viral **35, 40, 59, 91–92, 172**
Hepatitis
    Type A **44, 59, 102–103, 226**
    Type B **39, 59, 84–85, 112–113, 115–120, 139, 163–165, 214, 226**
    Type C **40, 60, 86–87, 112–113, 139, 167, 226**
    Delta **60, 86, 167, 226**
    Type E **44, 60, 102–103, 226**
    Type Non-A,Non-B **40, 60, 87, 112–113, 167**
Hepatitis B vaccine **85, 112–113, 140, 145, 149, 174**
Hepatitis B vaccine declination statement **149**
Herpangina **44, 60**
Herpes simplex **17, 35, 42, 60, 81, 103–104**
Herpes zoster **36, 42, 60**
Herpetic Whitlow **103**
High Risk Behavior **82, 174**
Histoplasmosis **61, 81, 226**
Hookworm disease **61**
Hot packs **131**
Housekeeping **143–145**
Human Immunodeficiency Virus – See HIV
ISG **112–113**
Immunization(s) **18, 145, 214**
Immunocompromised **18, 61**
Immunosuppressant **18, 61**
Impetigo **35, 61, 108, 109**
Incident reports **145**
Incubation period **17**
Indirect contact **17**
Infection **17, 157–159**
Infection control **21, 157–159**
Infectious diseases **157–159**
Infectious mononucleosis **61**
Influenza in infants and young children **35, 61, 226**
Insignia, uniform **220–221**
Intravenous (IV) fluids/poles **131**

Isolation **21, 33–74**
    AFB **33, 37**
    Blood/body fluid precautions **33, 39–40**
    Contact **33, 35–36**
    Drainage/secretion precautions **33, 41–42**
    Enteric precautions **33, 43–44**
    Respiratory **33, 37–38**
Isoniazid **110, 181, 183, 187**
Jakob-Creutzfeldt **39, 55, 61, 90, 171**
Jaundice **48**
Jewelry **221**
Jump suit **21, 29–30**
Kaposi's sarcoma **82**
Kawasaki syndrome **61**
Keratoconjunctivitis **42, 61**
Kwell **107**
Labels and signs **146**
Laryngitis – see pharyngitis
Laryngoscope **131**
Lassa fever **35, 61, 91–92, 172**
Legionella **65**
Legionnaires' disease **61**
Leprosy **61, 226**
Leptospirosis **40, 61, 92–93, 170, 226**
Lice **36, 95, 158, 171**
Linens **128–129, 131, 144**
Listeria monocytogenes meningitis **62**
Listeriosis **62**
Liver **84, 163, 164**
Lockjaw **109**
Lyme disease **62**
Lymphocytic choriomeningitis **62**
Lymphogranuloma **62**
MAST **132**
Magill forceps **131**
Malaria **18, 40, 62, 93–94, 168, 226**
Malta fever **53**

Marburg virus disease **35, 62, 91–92, 172**
Mask(s) **21, 26–28, 35, 37, 39, 41, 43**
Material safety data sheet(s) (MSDS) **128**
Measles **37, 62, 97, 121, 214, 227**
Medical records **148, 195–196, 198–201**
Mediterranean fever **91**
Melioidosis **62**
Meningitis **17, 36–37, 44, 62, 104–105, 227**
Meningococcal **17, 37, 63, 65, 104**
Meningococcemia **37, 63, 104**
Methods of compliance **140–141**
Microorganism **17**
Minocycline **104**
Molluscum contagiosus **63**
Moniliasis **53**
Monitor **132**
Monitoring **205–210**
Mononucleosis **61**
Mosquito-borne infections **18, 168**
Mucomycosis **63**
Multiple resistant organism **36, 63**
Multiple-resistant bacteria, infection or colonization **36, 63, 65**
Mumps **37, 63, 97–98, 214**
Mycobacterium leprae **42, 63**
Mycobacterium non TB **42, 63**
Mycoplasma pneumoniae **63, 65**
NIOSHA **162**
Nasal cannula **125, 132**
Nasopharyngeal airway **129**
Nebulizers **125, 132**
Necrotizing entercolitis **44, 64**
Needles and syringes **125–126, 132, 141**
Needlestick **112–113**
Needlestick panel **112–113**
Neisseria gonorrhea **62**
Neisseria meningitidis **62**
Neutropenia **64**

Nocardia asteroides **64**
Non-disposable equipment **127**
Nocardiosis **64**
Norwalk agent **44, 64**
OPIM **125, 141**
OSHA **115, 120, 139, 231**
OSHA state plan states **149**
Occupational exposure **139**
Orf **64**
Organism **17**
Oropharyngeal airway **125, 129**
Other potentially infectious material (OPIM) **125, 141**
Outerwear **21, 28, 29, 37, 39, 41, 43**
Oxygen delivery equipment **125, 132–133**
Oxygen extension tubing **125, 132**
PPE **25–32, 142–143, 173**
PTL tubes **133**
PR – see particulate respirator
Parainfluenza viruses **64**
Pediculosis **36, 64**
Penlight **133**
Percutaneous **85, 162, 164**
Personal protective equipment (PPE) **25–32 ,142–143, 173**
Personnel **217–218**
Pertussis (Whooping Cough) **37, 64, 72, 99, 227**
Pharngitis **36, 64, 69**
Pharyngeal diphtheria **35**
Phycomycosis **73**
Pillows **133**
Pink eye **48, 98**
Pinworm disease **57, 64**
Plague **36, 42, 64, 105–106, 227**
Pleurodynia **44, 64**
Pneumococcal meninigitis **63, 65**
Pneumocystis carinii **65, 81**
Pneumonia **36, 37, 42, 64, 65, 69, 81, 106, 227**
Pocket Masks **133**

Policy statements **79, 141, 217–222**
Poliomyelitis **44, 66, 227**
Poliovirus **66**
Post-exposure evaluation and follow-up **145–146**
Pre-employment physicals **213**
Precautions **33**
Psittacosis **66**
QA **205–210**
Q fever **66**
Quality assessment **207–208**
Quality Assurance **205–210**
Rabies **36, 66, 106–107, 227**
Rashes **48**
Rat-bite fever **40, 66**
Records **148, 195**
Recordkeeping **148, 193–204**
    Medical records **148, 195–196, 198–201**
    Training records **148, 197, 202–204**
Red measles **37, 62, 97, 122**
Regulated waste **125–126, 143–144**
Regulators, oxygen **125, 133**
Relapsing fever **40, 66, 92, 95–96, 171, 227**
Resistant bacterial infections **66**
Respiratory disease **66**
Respiratory infections, acute **35**
Respiratory isolation **33, 37–38**
Respiratory symptoms **48**
Respiratory syncytial viruses **66**
Restraints **133**
Resuscitator **133**
Reye's Syndrome **67**
Rheumatic fever **67**
Rhinoviruses **67**
Rickettsial fevers, tickborne **67**
Rickettsialpox **67**
Rifampin **110, 183, 187**
Ringworm **67**

Ritters' disease **67–78**
Rocky Mountain spotted fever **18, 67**
Roseola infantum **67**
Rotavirus **58, 67**
Rubella **36, 55, 59, 67, 98–99, 214**
Rubeola – see measles
Salmonella **18, 44, 58, 107**
Salmonellosis **58, 67, 227**
Sandbags **133**
Scabies **36, 68, 107, 227**
Scalded skin syndrome **36, 67, 68**
Scarlet fever **69**
Schistosomiasis **68**
Scissors **133**
Sharps **125–126, 141**
Sharps containers **126, 141**
Shigella **44, 58, 108**
Shigellosis **58, 68, 227**
Shingles – see also herpes zoster, varicella zoster **36, 42, 60**
Signs **146**
Skin infections **36, 41**
Skin tests, TB **177–179**
Sleeve protection **31**
Smallpox **36, 68, 228**
Sore throat **36**
Spirillium minus disease **68**
Splints **134**
Sporotrichosis **68**
Spotted fever, Rocky Mountain **18, 67**
Squad bench **134**
Staphylococcal **42, 43, 58, 65, 68, 108**
Sterile equipment **134**
Sterilization **127**
Stethoscope **134**
Straps **134**
Streptobacillus **69**
Streptococcal **42, 58, 69, 109, 228**

Streptococcus pneumonia **65, 69**
Stretcher **131, 134**
Strict isolation **33, 35–36**
Strongyloidiasis **69**
Stylets **134**
Suction equipment **134**
Suits **29**
Surveillance **205–210**
Susceptible host **17–18**
Symbols **46–48, 50–73**
Syphilis **40, 42, 72, 94–95, 167**
Symptom specific isolation **45–48**
Tapeworm **70**
Tetanus **70, 109–110, 214, 228**
Thermometers **135**
Thrush **53**
Tinea **70**
Tongue blades **135**
Toxic shock syndrome **42, 68, 70**
Toxoplasmosis **70, 81**
Trachoma, acute **42, 70**
Trachomatis **42**
Training **147–148, 159–190**
    General infection control **157–159**
    Exposure control plans for bloodborne pathogens **159–174**
    Tuberculosis **174–184**
    Records **148, 197, 202–204**
Transmission of infectious agents **17–18, 175–176**
    Airborne **18, 175–176**
    Contact **17**
    Droplet **17**
    Indirect contact **17**
    Vectorborne **18**
    Vehicle **18**
Transport **75–76**
Trench fever **70, 228**
Trichinosis **70**

Index

Trichomoniasis **71**
Trichuriasis **71**
Trousers, MAST **132**
Tuberculocidal **39, 127, 129–135**
Tuberculosis **18, 37, 42, 71, 110–111, 174–190, 192, 215–216**
    TB meningitis **63**
    TB skin testing **177**
    TB screening **215–216**
    TB treatment **179–184, 187–190**
Tularemia **42, 71**
Typhoid Fever **44, 71, 228**
Typhus **71, 228**
Ulcers **41**
Undulant fever – See brucellosis
Uniforms **220**
Universal Precautions **23, 24, 125, 173**
Urinals **135**
Urinary tract infection **71**
Vaccine **145**
Vaccinia **36, 71**
Varicella **36, 72**
Varicella – Zoster virus **36, 42, 60, 82, 92**
Variola **72**
Vector **18**
Vector-borne transmission **18**
Vehicle transmission **18**
Venezuelan equine encephalitis **52**
Vibrio parahaemolyticus, gastroenteritis **44, 59, 72**
Vincent's angina **72**
Viral pneumonia **66, 72**
Viral encephalitis **52**
Viral pericarditis, myocarditis, meningitis **44, 72**
Viral hemorrhagic fever **35, 40, 59, 91–92, 172**
Vomit **48**
Western equine encephalitis **52**
Whitlow, herpetic **103**
Whooping cough **37, 64, 72, 99**

Work practice controls **141–142, 173**
Wound infections **36, 41, 72, 111**
Yaws **72**
Yellow fever **72**
Yersinia entercolitica **44, 59, 72**
Yersiniosis **59**
Zoster **36, 42, 73**
Zygomycosis **73**

NOTES

NOTES

NOTES

NOTES

NOTES

NOTES